Somatic Therapy for Healing Trauma

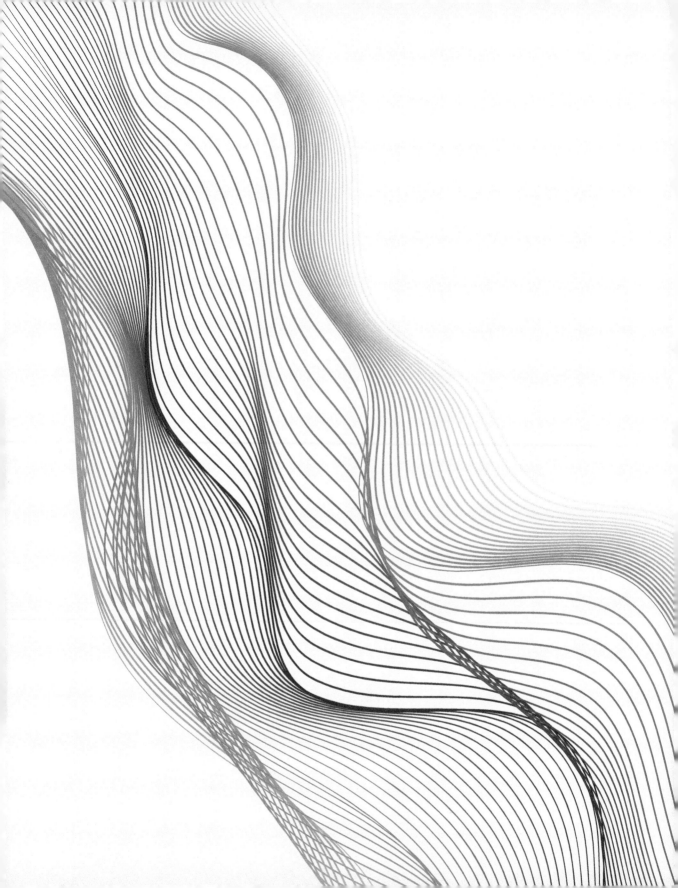

SOMATIC THERAPY
for Healing Trauma

Effective Tools
to Strengthen the
Mind-Body Connection

JORDAN DANN, LP

ROCKRIDGE
PRESS

This book is dedicated to the teachers throughout my life who have helped me develop and nurture a relationship with my body.

First Rockridge Press trade paperback edition 2022

For general information on our other products and services, please contact our Customer Care Department within the United States at (866) 744-2665, or outside the United States at (510) 253-0500.

Paperback ISBN: 978-1-68539-377-9 | eBook ISBN: 978-1-68539-996-2

Manufactured in the United States of America

Graphic Designer: Jarod Denmark
Interior and Cover Designer: Heather Krakora
Art Producer: Hannah Dickerson
Editor: Adrian Potts
Production Editor: Ashley Polikoff
Production Manager: David Zapanta

Illustrations used under license from Shutterstock.com on the following: pp. 17, 49, 82. Author photo courtesy of Will O'Hare.

10 9 8 7 6 5 4 3 2 1 0

Contents

Introduction

For several decades, psychology has focused on treating conditions like trauma through the mind alone. Perhaps, like so many clients when they first walk through my door, you have sought to treat your symptoms and challenges through conventional means but feel like there's still a missing piece in your healing.

Learning that memories, experiences, and emotions are stored not just in the mind but also the body opens up a new pathway to healing for many of my clients. This, in essence, is what somatic therapy strives to do—and what the information and tools in this book are designed to help you achieve.

When I first started my own process of healing and personal development in therapy, I was in my early thirties. Although I had some wonderful therapists and gained a lot of insight about my history, there continued to be a missing piece for me. One morning as I sat in my therapist's office, I thought to myself, "What about my body? We never talk about what's happening in my body."

My first career was as an actor and a singer, and then a teacher of voice and movement for actors. The overall aim of voice and movement training is to help actors awaken new connections between the voice, body, and mind through a process of physical awareness, imagery, breath work, and the progressive release of physical tension. As I began training actors and working directly with students' bodies, what I repeatedly encountered with my students was somatic memory and unprocessed trauma. As students worked in a safe environment with my support, and often the support of a group of other students, they became more aware of tension in their bodies. They were then able to release that tension, allowing them to let go of memories and experiences that had been directing their day-to-day experience. At a certain point, coaching actors for theatrical purposes began to feel like an interruption to the more essential healing process that I was interested in, and that is when I became a psychoanalyst.

Somatic focus has been the fundamental aspect of my own therapeutic journey, and I have worked with hundreds of individuals who have said that talk therapy wasn't enough; it was the incorporation of a somatic practice that finally changed their relationships with themselves.

This book is intended to help you work through any life transitions you might be experiencing. With that said, if you have ongoing physical health symptoms or suffer from debilitating anxiety and depression, you should seek out a medical professional. This book is not a replacement for therapy, medication, or medical treatment.

How to Use This Book

This workbook will offer you foundational knowledge of somatic therapy and provide experiential exercises for you to move through at your own pace that will deepen your relationship with your body and support your process of healing and self-development. If you are just embarking on learning more about your relationship to your body, or if you are working with a therapist and want to deepen and enhance your own therapy, this book is for you.

Part 1 of the workbook will offer you an introduction to somatic therapy, provide a brief history of somatic therapy, explore how somatic therapy addresses trauma and other symptoms, explain the different types of somatic therapy, and teach you the fundamental concepts of somatic therapy techniques. Part 2 of the workbook will build off the information provided in part 1, but depending on your needs, interests, or time constraints, feel free to create your own relationship with this workbook and skip around to explore the content that is most relevant or interesting to you.

Each chapter in part 2 includes education about key psychological concepts, along with corresponding practices, exercises, and affirmations to enhance your somatic therapy tool kit. A practice is something you can do outside of this book; exercises are activities to explore within the pages in this workbook; and affirmations are expressions of support to cheer you along in your somatic exploration. Feel free to write affirmations on sticky notes and post them around your living space or send yourself calendar reminders on your phone throughout the day. Affirmations are a wonderful way to internalize a supportive relationship with yourself as you develop these new skills and practices.

I am my body. My body is me.

PART I

Understanding Somatic Therapy

Somatic therapy is a growing field that moves beyond talk therapy to include the "felt experience" of a person in order to create an integrated treatment of the body, mind, and spirt, viewed as a functional whole. This approach to therapy, sometimes referred to as "bottom-up therapy," takes advantage of the brain's capacity for neuroplasticity and seeks to process traumatic memory and create new experiences of safety, resourcefulness, and vitality.

Somatic therapies address physical injuries, grief, trauma, anxiety, depression, and chronic pain through various techniques, including bringing attention to physical awareness, exploration of movement, use of imagery, breath work, bodywork, and touch.

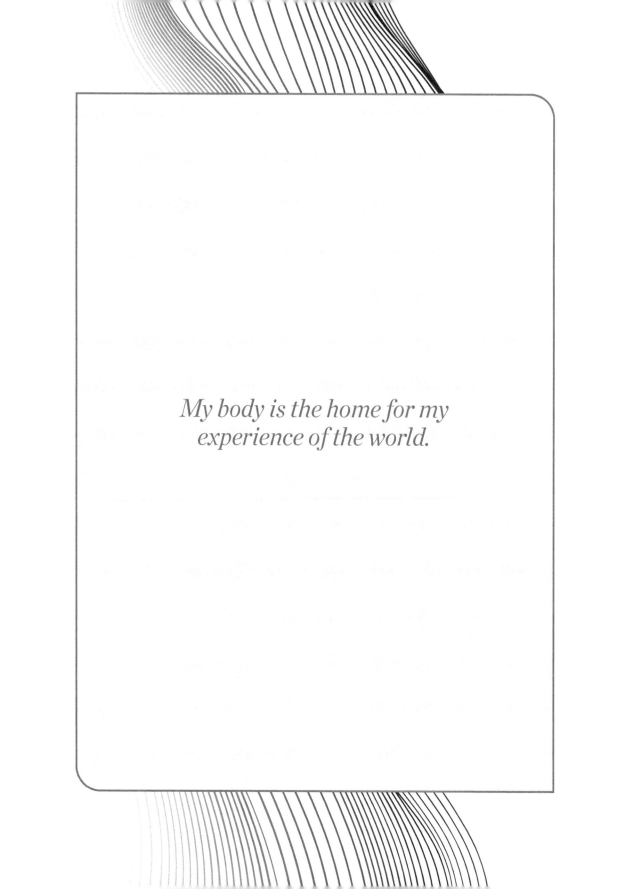

My body is the home for my experience of the world.

CHAPTER ONE

An Introduction to Somatic Therapy

Most of the world prioritizes thinking, but your head is only about 10 percent of your body weight. So what about the other 90 percent of your body? Somatic therapy is the practice of being mindfully aware of sensations in the body and learning how to regulate your body's nervous system when you are experiencing stress or other intense sensations. Somatic awareness is a skill you can learn.

When you experience symptoms such as anxiety, depression, emotional dysregulation, panic attacks, exhaustion, insomnia, and loss of appetite, they occur not only in the mind but also in the body. When you work with the body, you can release survival impulses and energy (such as fight, flight, or freeze responses) that may have become stuck, which can often address the root cause of the physical symptom. Working directly with your physical experience can support you in developing an increased tolerance for uncomfortable somatic sensations and increase your window of tolerance for the universal range of human emotion.

In the following chapter, you will learn what somatic therapy is, explore a brief history of somatic therapy, identify symptoms and issues that can be treated with somatic therapy, learn about the various modalities of somatic therapy, and deepen your understanding of the mind-body connection.

What Is Somatic Therapy?

Somatic psychotherapy focuses on restoring self-regulation of the autonomic nervous system, the body's "control system." The autonomic nervous system acts unconsciously and controls bodily functions such as breathing, heart rate, digestion, respiratory rate, eyesight, urination, and sexual arousal. Somatic therapy helps relieve emotional and physical stress that can become trapped in the autonomic nervous system as a result of trauma, chronic stressors, or other environmental conditions.

Somatic therapy is an evidence-based model of therapy and is sometimes referred to as "body therapy" or "bottom-up therapy." It is a way of sensing and exploring one's physical experience, and it can be integrated into any therapeutic approach. In addition to exploring thoughts and feelings, somatic therapy includes cultivating a connection to bodily sensation, movement, gestures, self-touch, and imagery.

Somatic therapy integrates current research in neuroscience, anatomy, physiology, and Eastern and Western practices and theories. It is more than just a skill set or practice; it is a path toward living an embodied and present-centered life. Whether you are coming to this workbook to address a singular traumatic event that occurred at any point in your life or you are hoping to address attachment trauma from your childhood, the approach and benefit are the same.

A Brief History of Somatic Therapy

The understanding that emotional and physical health are interlinked dates back to second-century physician Galen. In the twentieth century, Wilhelm Reich carried this concept forward with his 1933 book, *Character Analysis*. In this text, he introduced the concept of "body armor," exploring how repressed emotions can affect muscular tension, body posture, and physical movement.

In the 1950s, the philosopher Eugene Gendlin introduced the concept of "felt-sense," which describes the ability to sense emotional experiences in the body rather than solely in the mind. This was an influential concept for the work of Peter Levine, who, in the 1970s, developed a pioneering approach called "somatic experiencing"—a body-oriented approach to the healing of trauma and other stress disorders.

Somatic Therapy in the Modern Age

In recent decades, there has been a steady shift away from the idea that the mind and body are separate entities. This is thanks in large part to the work of Peter Levine, Bessel van der Kolk, and others who brought somatic psychology into the mainstream, specifically in regard to trauma. Over the past thirty years, empirical evidence in neuroscience, medical science, and psychology have come into alignment: There is no real division between the body and the brain.

Today, somatic approaches are used in a number of fields, including psychology, meditation, art, movement, dance, and bodywork. It moves beyond talk therapy to include the "felt experience" of a person in their body as a primary means of understanding what is going on in the mind.

Somatic Therapy and Trauma

Trauma begins as intense stress to the nervous system from a perceived life-threat or as the cumulative result of ongoing stress. Both types of stress can seriously impair the ability to function with optimal health. Trauma can result from a broad range of stressful stimuli, such as sexual and physical abuse, emotional abuse, neglect, accidents, invasive medical procedures, war, natural disasters, immigration, birth trauma, loss, discrimination, or any other number of stresses that result in ongoing fear, boundary intrusion, or conflict.

When faced with a threatening stimulus, the sympathetic nervous system, the branch of the autonomic nervous system that prepares the body for immediate action, triggers the body's fight, flight, freeze, or fawn response. When it is working best, the sympathetic nervous system scans the environment and is able to correctly assess when there is a threat and respond as needed. When the threatening stimulus is gone, the parasympathetic nervous system comes online and the body moves into relaxation, or "rest and digest" mode. This collaboration and exchange between the sympathetic and parasympathetic nervous systems supports blood pressure, breathing rate, hormone flow, and a return to homeostasis.

Any type of event or stimulus that the body perceives as threatening pushes the nervous system outside its ability to self-regulate. For some people who experience trauma, the system gets stuck in the "on" position, which can result in an ongoing sense of danger, overstimulation, and an inability to relax.

Somatic therapy helps people who have experienced trauma become more aware of sensations in the body and learn to use therapeutic techniques to begin to rebalance the autonomic nervous system, bringing individuals out of the feedback loop of the past and into the here and now. The tools in this book are designed to achieve this.

Applications of Somatic Therapy

Somatic therapy releases traumatic shock, which is key to transforming many psychological and psychical symptoms. Somatic therapy offers a framework to assess where a person is stuck in the fight, flight, or freeze response and to provide clinical tools and interpersonal support to resolve these fixed physiological autonomic nervous system states. "Stuck" looks different for each individual and is dependent upon an individual's encounter with the traumatic stimulus or repeated stimuli experienced.

Somatic therapy is used to treat a range of conditions, including PTSD, C-PTSD, anxiety, depression, grief, and chronic pain.

PTSD and C-PTSD

Post-traumatic stress disorder (PTSD) and complex post-traumatic stress disorder (C-PTSD) are both mental health conditions that develop after experiencing a traumatic event. The difference between the two conditions is the frequency and duration of the trauma and resulting symptoms.

At the core of post-traumatic experience is a somatic state of nervous system overwhelm. When overwhelm occurs, your ability to be present with many aspects of your experience checks out, and your sensory experience becomes fractured into disparate associated elements: emotion, behavior, affect, thought, instinct, image, and sensation.

The human brain can process eleven million bits of information every second, but your conscious mind can handle only forty to fifty bits of information per second. When you experience something that you perceive as a threat, your body responds by moving into survival mode in order to protect you. However, research bears out that much of the other millions of bits of information that you take in during the traumatic event stay in the body as implicit memory. An implicit memory can leave us feeling triggered by things we aren't fully aware of or that don't make sense to us, yet that we have big emotional reactions to. For example, if a person was hit by a car outside of a coffee shop, months or even years later the smell of coffee might trigger a panic attack because the scent is interpreted as a sign of danger.

It might be helpful to think of trauma as something that fragments your sense of self and somatic therapy as something that invites fragmentation to come back into awareness, allowing for recovery and reintegration of those parts of yourself and of your experience that have been out of awareness.

Anxiety and Depression

An anxious state can be thought of as the sympathetic nervous system being stuck in the fight position. In this state, it is common to feel nervous, restless, tense, agitated, frustrated, angry, or vigilant to perceived threats to your safety. A depressed state can be thought of as the parasympathetic nervous system being stuck in the freeze position. In this state, it is common to feel sad, apathetic, hopeless, fatigued, or dissociated. Both states are accompanied by negative thoughts that can repeat on a loop.

You might think of somatic therapy like going to the gym for your nervous system. A healthy nervous system is flexible and can move back and forth between parasympathetic and sympathetic responses. Somatic therapy uses a variety of exercises to bring flexibility back to your physiological state so that your nervous system is responsive to the present context, as opposed to the threat or overwhelm from the past.

Grief

When you experience the loss of a supportive relationship, your nervous system becomes disoriented and you need to assist your nervous system to reorient or rebalance the geography of your body with new resources and supports.

There are different kinds of grief. If a relationship with a romantic partner comes to an end, it may bring up unprocessed grief connected to the loss of a parent. Grief becomes unprocessed when you receive little compassion, understanding, or support to help you reorganize and reorient to the world. Somatic therapy serves to support someone's process of grieving and develop new resources of connection.

Chronic Pain

Chronic physical pain is initially sensed in the body through nociceptors, the sensory receptors at the end of sensory neurons specifically organized to send pain signals to the spinal cord and brain. If you have a history of feeling physical pain, you might contract or tense your body to prepare for the anticipated sensation. You may also have associated negative thoughts or narratives about what the pain means or what it says about who you are. These factors can induce a state of high arousal in the nervous system, which can lead to patterns that end up causing more pain.

Somatic therapy helps develop awareness about the intricacies of this process and supports your system to move into more relaxed states or accept your physical experience in a new way that makes pain symptoms less severe.

Understanding the Mind-Body Connection

Somatic therapy invites you to consider a holistic approach to well-being that involves bringing your mind and body into balance to create harmony and health. This modality helps you become aware of how trauma manifests in the body and explore ideas to release it, which can in turn benefit your emotional well-being. A healthy mind is a mind that can be aware of the body, notice when there are overwhelming feelings of stress, fear, and worry, and make choices to respond in a way that restores a sense of equanimity and peace.

You may also see the term "mind-body-spirit connection." This introduces a third element in the form of the human "spirit." For some, this may be a spiritual conception of the human soul, while for others, this may simply refer to being a part of a community, having a connection to the natural world, or cultivating qualities such as presence, gratitude, joy, hope, positivity, and connection.

Somatic therapy pioneer Peter Levine has noted that in trauma situations, the brain acts in two ways that create two different states of being: "survival brain" or "safe brain." In safe brain, you are able to be in the present moment and you are open to taking in new information, tolerating ambiguity, and having expansive awareness. You feel calm, peaceful, curious, and safe. When survival brain is activated, the fear center of the brain is lit up and you become hyper-focused, feel threatened, and cannot tolerate ambiguity. Fear dominates decision-making, and you do not feel safe. All of your life energy is used on "protecting" you from danger that is no longer present. If you have experienced trauma, you might be living in survival brain, which depletes your vitality and results in a diminished capacity to live. Somatic therapy aims to gradually release and redirect this energy so that you can move into safe brain.

Healing Is Possible with Somatic Therapy

Renowned trauma therapist Bessel van der Kolk writes, "Traumatized people chronically feel unsafe inside their bodies: The past is alive in the form of gnawing interior discomfort." When you experience trauma, your body is constantly being sent signals that you are still under threat, and, in an attempt to control these uncomfortable thoughts and sensations, you can become an expert at ignoring your gut feelings. This adaptive process can mean that you numb yourself, and over time, this can mean a loss of identity and a loss of your sense of connectedness to others and the world in which you are living.

When the body holds traumatic memory, you can get stuck in chronic trauma responses of fight, flight, freeze, or fawn in the body, which cause a variety of issues in your body and mind. The reason somatic therapy has the potential to help traumatized individuals more than a cognitive (mind-focused) approach is that when you start to become aware of your somatic experience, your body and mind begin to create a sense of internal safety.

Whether you are experiencing physical or psychological symptoms, processing trauma, or just wanting to deepen your mind-body-spirit connection, working with your somatic awareness will support your ability to be aware of what you feel and make choices to bring your body back into ease and regulation.

Key Takeaways

In this chapter, you've learned about the basics of somatic therapy and how it can help heal trauma in your body and improve your overall well-being.

- Somatic therapy helps you find awareness of the physical sensations inside your body.

- The more awareness you have about your physical sensations, the more you support your ability to address psychological and physical symptoms, process trauma, and become more integrated in your thoughts, feelings, and bodily sensations.

- One of the underlying theories of somatic therapy is that your body's memory of the trauma is more important than your cognitive memory. Somatic therapy is a bottom-up form of therapy that works directly with the autonomic nervous system to release unprocessed trauma, stress, and tension.

I feel, therefore I am.

Beginning Your Somatic Therapy Journey

In the following chapter you'll learn more about how somatic therapy works and what its key techniques are and become acquainted with various forms of somatic therapy. While somatic therapy is a form of therapy, it is important to understand that it isn't just a tool or a strategy; it's a path to living an embodied life. When you learn to listen to your body, you can move into greater vitality with an increased capacity to move toward what you want and away from what you don't want. Somatic therapy is a path toward healing and also a process of developing a lifelong friendship with the nearest environment you have: your body.

Your abilities to notice, sense, and feel are the foundational skills of somatic therapy. The more you can listen to what your body is telling you, the more equipped you will be to meet your needs as they arise. As you move through this workbook and begin to incorporate the various exercises and practices into your life, it is really important that you repeat all the skills you are learning. Repetition is crucial when it comes to learning and incorporating new ways of being and unlearning other responses that no longer serve you.

How Somatic Therapy Works

Somatic therapy works to restore optimal health and flexibility to the autonomic nervous system. This is the part of your nervous system that controls involuntary actions, like your heart rate and breathing.

In simple terms, the autonomic nervous system operates like a car. It can either press the gas pedal to create more energy or use the brake pedal to slow down or stop. This occurs in its two main parts: the sympathetic nervous system, which increases energy and arousal (gas), and the parasympathetic nervous system, which helps you slow down and come into calmer, less-aroused states (brake).

You grew up in a particular environment or environments and had unique experiences that shaped your nervous system. The way your nervous system was shaped has a direct impact on your physical health, as well as on your capacity to cope with emotions and respond to stress. Some may be able to easily engage the gas pedal of their nervous system but may not have easy access to the brake pedal.

Dan Siegel coined the term "window of tolerance," which is the zone in which people are able to stay calm and rational when they encounter challenges. Somatic therapy aims to widen this window of tolerance so that you can better manage the ups and downs of life.

Understanding Trauma

When it comes to understanding trauma, many in the field of somatic therapy advocate for a strengths-based approach. Rather than seeing trauma as a negative label, a problem, or something that is wrong with you, you can choose to see it as your natural effort to persevere in spite of life's challenges. This allows you to see beyond labels or limitations placed on you by yourself and others and to instead acknowledge and build upon your strengths.

Trauma is not what happened to you or who you are; rather, it's what your body carries as the imprint of what happened to you. Trauma is also what you hold inside as a result of not having another empathetic and compassionate person to witness your pain. *Trauma is part of the human experience.* Trauma is not the story of what has happened to one person; it is what each person experiences throughout a lifetime, in some form or another. It is a cultural phenomenon, a global phenomenon, and you are a part of the human experience.

Trauma is a way that you seek safety. It is your body's adaptive brilliance that becomes maladaptive unless you learn to attend to your body. If you don't learn to listen to your body and you don't befriend your nervous system, trauma can take away your vitality and keep you stuck in ways of being that no longer serve you.

Emotional Trauma

Emotional trauma is the end result of events or experiences that leave you feeling unsafe, helpless, and alone. Emotional trauma can result from a single event or a period of prolonged or ongoing experiences, such as abuse, neglect, bullying, discrimination, or humiliation. When this occurs in childhood and results in the disruption of the bond between a child and parent, it is otherwise known as attachment trauma.

Emotional trauma is recognizable by a persistent sense of danger, uneasiness, or anxiety. It can also result in depression and physical symptoms such as insomnia, nightmares, or other health conditions. Somatic therapy aims to identify the somatic sensations associated with developmental trauma and to begin to expand the window of tolerance to reestablish balance in the nervous system.

Physical Trauma

Physical trauma, or traumatic injury, is a term that refers to physical injuries of sudden onset and severity that require immediate medical attention. Physical trauma can cause systemic shock called "shock trauma." Physical trauma may be caused by various forces from outside the body, including falls, traffic accidents, drowning, assaults, burns, and both invasive and noninvasive surgery.

Research has demonstrated that chronic pain may be caused by not only physical injury but also the ongoing emotional and neurological impact of thoughts and feelings about the pain. People who have experienced trauma and suffer from PTSD are often at a higher risk for developing chronic pain. During a traumatic event, the nervous system goes into survival mode and sometimes has difficulty moving back toward relaxation and a feeling of safety. If the nervous system doesn't come back into balance, this can result in high activity of stress hormones, which increases blood pressure and changes blood levels. Over time, this can reduce the immune system's ability to heal.

A Note on the Approach to Physical Touch

Touch is the first language you experience in life, so it is natural when working in the nonverbal realm to consider it. Good touch delivers sensations to your brain that release oxytocin, the "cuddle hormone" that plays a key role in helping you bond with others and feel safe, and other "feel-good" hormones. These neurochemical changes make you feel happier and calmer, lower your heart rate, ease muscle tension, and support breathing, sleep, digestion, and immune response.

Physical touch has long been a controversial issue in psychotherapy, and it is widely believed that touch can be too easily misunderstood or abused and can cause adverse reactions in patients that can harm the therapeutic relationship and interrupt treatment. For those who have experienced physical or sexual trauma, touch can sometimes induce re-traumatization or damage the therapeutic alliance between client and practitioner. Many somatic therapists are trained and certified to offer touch as an intervention and support to healing trauma. If you are interested in touch as a component to your healing process, seek out practitioners who have engaged in this degree of training and certification.

While this workbook does not include physical touch exercises or interventions, the uses of self-touch and therapeutic touch by a licensed practitioner have proven to be widely beneficial. Many alternative, body-centered therapies include physical touch and have been an important aspect of healing and recovery for many. These interventions include massage therapy, the Feldenkrais Method, Rolfing, reflexology, acupuncture, the Alexander Technique, and dance or movement therapy.

Key Somatic Therapy Techniques

The governing theory across somatic therapy modalities involves "neuroplasticity," which is the brain's ability to change and adapt as a result of experience. Somatic therapy modalities also include a process of working with your physical experience as a way to rebalance your nervous system and create new neurological pathways that bring you out of various repetitive negative "loops" of the past and into more positive feelings in the present.

Neuroplasticity research has become increasingly popular over the past decade, and it has become clear that the brain has the capacity to adapt and change, a process referred to as "neurogenesis." Neural pathways in the brain are strengthened with repetition, and a common phrase used to capture this concept is "Neurons that fire together, wire together." Constant repetition of an experience, either in the instance of attachment or developmental trauma or in the case of "retriggering" as a result of shock trauma, means that these neurological patterns and the resulting behavior can become more fixed.

Somatic therapies incorporate techniques to build new neurological pathways that move traumatic experience from "implicit memory" (always happening) to "explicit memory" (happened in the past) and aim to support a felt and perceived experience of safety in the present.

In later chapters you will be offered a general introduction to these key somatic therapy concepts and techniques. This psychology education and the exercises in this book will allow you to begin to practice a new way of thinking about traumatic experience that will hopefully support your capacity to move toward increased awareness of the sensations in your body as well as how to create increased feelings of safety inside your body.

Body Awareness

Body awareness and the felt-sense are key terms in somatic therapy. Body awareness is when you focus your awareness on internal body sensations. Body awareness is an inherent aspect of embodied self-awareness that supports identity, relationality, and choice—all of which are paramount to your sense of self. Additionally, body awareness is key to your ability to sense what you need and feel so that you can make clear choices about what you want (or don't want) in your life.

Grounding

Grounding is a somatic approach that refers to a person's ability to experience themselves through their physical presence. The purpose of grounding is to support "proprioception," which is your ability to sense your movement, action, and location. Grounding focuses on your ability to sense the support of the earth, or the support of the chair beneath you, or the orientation of things within the space around you—all in service of regulating your nervous system. Grounding practices are a key resource for trauma recovery and can help you manage sensations of emotional overwhelm and physical pain.

Pendulation

Pendulation is the natural movement between states of expansion and states of contraction that occur in your nervous system. Pendulation is a basic principle of organic life, seen in the ebb and flow of ocean tides, the motion of bird wings, and the cycle of seasons. A resilient nervous system is one that can move back and forth between alert action and rest and digest without getting stuck at either extreme. Pendulation also introduces "resourced" (safe) states to develop confidence in your nervous system to move between inverse states.

Titration

Titration is the concept of "less is more"—the precept that working slowly, and with small amounts of traumatic experience or sensation, is a safe and gradual way to process and renegotiate trauma. The "trauma vortex" is a metaphor that describes the whirlpool of overwhelming sensations and emotions that are often a result of traumatic experience. Titration is an inherent aspect of the "healing vortex"—the counterbalance that supports the mastery, choice, and resourcefulness that are a part of healing.

Sequencing

Sequencing is a somatic-based process of your body releasing stored tension resulting from trauma. Sequencing can be thought of as a chain reaction. For example, tension in the belly may begin to move upward, or lightness in the arms might turn to heaviness. Sequencing may also bring up other forms of release. You may cry as a way of letting go of emotions, or laugh as you feel more powerful. Each body is different, and each person will move through a sequencing process in their own way.

Resourcing

When trauma gets stuck in your nervous system, even though the event is over, every time you encounter an associated stimulus or trigger, your evolutionary brain, which is concerned with survival, trips an alarm system that registers as "danger." Resourcing is a process of inviting your mind-body to attune to sensations of safety that are available in the present moment. The process of attending to a feeling of safety teaches your nervous system that it can experience stress and then return to a state of calm. There are infinite ways to resource, a few of which include grounding, affirmations, nourishing relationships, and creative imagery.

The following is designed to help you start turning your awareness inside your body and noticing how it feels right now. This will be a key skill used throughout the book. Find a comfortable position and close your eyes. Make note of which muscles or areas of your body feel tense or contracted. Note also which areas of your body feel relaxed or pleasant. Make circles, marks, and notes on the body illustration of any awareness you have of sensations of tension or relaxation.

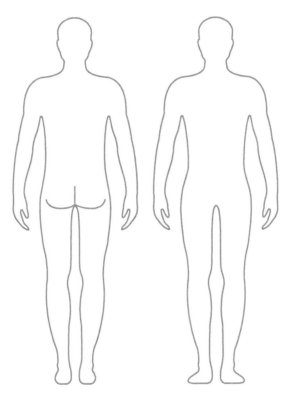

You may notice that you have "hot spots" in your body where you regularly notice tension. You may also notice that there are reliable areas inside your body where you regularly experience feelings of ease. If you are able to identify these areas, make a note on your illustration.

Don't worry if you find it challenging to observe what sensations arise; you'll have many more opportunities to develop this skill throughout the book. For the moment, give yourself space to begin noticing whatever comes up.

When to Seek Guidance from a Somatic Therapist

If you suffer from ongoing depression, relationship issues, anxiety, obsessive thinking, substance use, or any other cognitive or behavioral issues that interrupt your day-to-day functioning, then you should consult a therapist to see if psychological or psychiatric treatment is right for you. Even people who experience milder symptoms find therapy to be beneficial and supportive. The benefit of working with a somatic therapist is that you will be offered support, containment, and ongoing psychoeducation as you embark on healing or self-development.

Researchers have found that the therapeutic alliance between therapist and client is what plays the greatest role in effectiveness of treatment. Therefore, what is most important is that you pay attention to your own responses as you interview providers and ask questions about their therapeutic approach. No matter how much professional experience someone has, what is most important is your feeling of comfort, safety, and trust.

Key Takeaways

Somatic therapy is rooted in somatic psychology—a body-mind-spirt approach to psychology. Somatic therapy aims to address the feedback loop that runs continually between the mind and the body. Somatic therapy differs from traditional talk therapy, as the focus is on somatic experience, sensation, movement, and behavior arising from the body.

- A shared theory among most forms of somatic therapy is that traumatic experience stays trapped in the body and, through various somatic interventions, this trapped experience can be released, thus restoring regulation to the autonomic nervous system.

- Dan Siegel coined the term "window of tolerance," which describes the zone somatic therapy aims to expand in order to support greater effectiveness and health.

- Many forms of somatic therapy aim to move traumatic experience from implicit memory (still happening) to explicit memory (happened in the past).

- Most somatic therapy modalities include the following techniques: body awareness, grounding, pendulation, titration, sequencing, and resourcing.

*I grant myself the space and curiosity
to get to know my body and listen
to what it has to teach me.*

PART II

Your Somatic Therapy Tool Kit

The next six chapters will center on key somatic therapy techniques. Each chapter will provide a bit of psycho-education as well as positive affirmations, prompts, practices, and exercises to support your embodiment journey. Positive affirmations are statements that you can repeat to yourself to support your learning, instill positive thoughts, and combat negative thinking. Prompts are intended to deepen and expand theoretical concepts. Practices are activities for you to explore outside of the book to support the incorporation of concepts, and exercises are activities for you to explore inside the book.

Remember that the most important part of learning something new or developing new habits is repetition—especially since somatic therapy is about working to change habitual patterns in your body and mind. Feel free to jump around the chapters to the exercises that you feel drawn toward and repeat the exercises or practices that feel good for you. Sometimes somatic work can feel difficult, tiring, or bring up a lot of emotions when you first begin, so remember to take breaks when that is what your body is telling you to do.

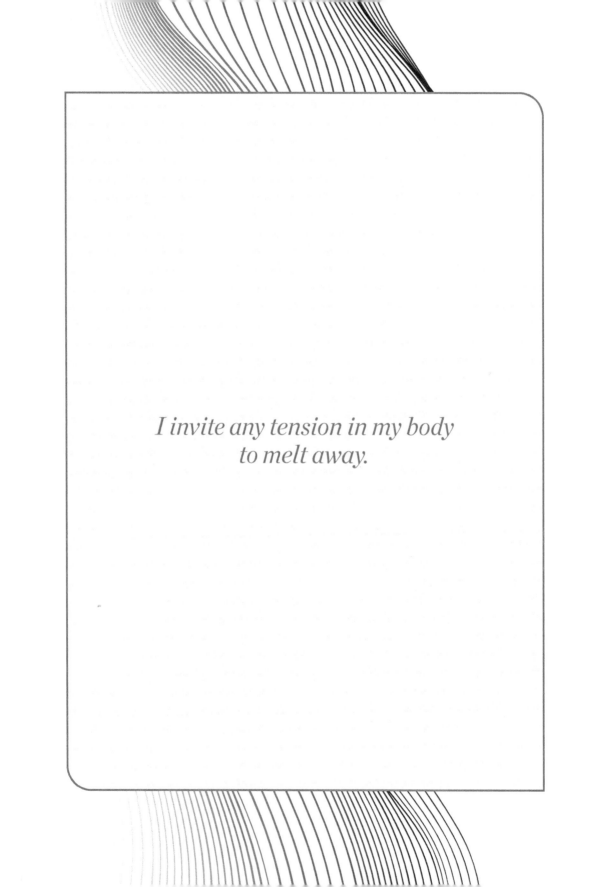

*I invite any tension in my body
to melt away.*

CHAPTER THREE

Releasing Tension with Body Awareness Tools

Two of the most important things you can do for your overall health and well-being are learning to become aware of tension and learning to release tension with relaxation. Chronic stress and physical tension have been referred to as "silent killers," as they compromise the immune system and can have a serious impact on your day-to-day mood and functioning. They are increasingly recognized by the scientific and medical community as a major contributor to persistent and chronic disease, such as heart disease, gastrointestinal problems, and sleep disorders.

In this chapter you will explore the process of saying hello to all the parts of your body so that you can begin to notice what your felt experience is throughout the whole of your body. You will also learn an essential skill called "tracking," which is a process of examining the sensations you are experiencing in your body in the present moment. And you will develop language for describing sensations of tension and relaxation, explore breathing that supports relaxation, and engage in exercises that support your ability to release tension.

Putting Body Awareness into Practice

Encountering stress is a normal part of being human, and when you encounter stress, it's normal for your body to constrict. When you carry chronic tension, it can begin to wear down your body, resulting in long-term consequences such as anxiety, depression, weight gain, poor sleep, physical pain, and bad posture.

Every person holds tension in their body differently. You may notice tension in your jaw, shoulders, chest, stomach, legs, or hands. Bring your curiosity to your body as you begin to track what kinds of things cause tension in your body and where you feel the tension when you experience stressful stimuli.

As you develop physical awareness, you will begin to notice when your body constricts with tension, and you will gradually be able to self-direct to bring relaxation and release to your body.

Physical awareness and relaxation techniques take practice and consistency. In time you will be able to use these tools in any moment to de-stress and change your state of being.

Take a moment to think about a time when you felt really relaxed. You might think of a special place that you like to visit in nature, or some relaxing place in your home. You can also use your imagination to create a place that feels relaxing to you. Take a few moments to close your eyes and notice the details of this place. Then shift your awareness to how you feel in your body as you imagine this place. In the space below, describe the relaxing image in your mind, how you feel in your body as you imagine it, and any thoughts that come up.

Take a moment to think about the last time you experienced something stressful. Maybe you had an encounter with a neighbor, coworker, or a partner that created some tension in your body. Now, close your eyes and notice where you feel tension in the body as you bring the memory to mind. When you are ready, write about what came to mind as you reflected on the event. Make note also of where you observed tension in your body as you reflected on the event.

BODY SCAN

The following practice is a foundational practice of somatic therapy. Body scanning is something that you can do in any context, at any time of day, to support your awareness. Body scanning is a primary way in which you can receive information from your body that can become an essential part of helping you tune in to what you are feeling or needing in any given moment. You might think of somatic awareness as a helpful way to stay "up to date" with yourself.

1. Find a comfortable position, either sitting or lying down. Feel free to allow your eyes to gently close. If you prefer to have them open, you can allow a soft gaze, cast downward.

2. Notice your breath moving in and out of your body. Feel the air coming in through your mouth or nose and then releasing out.

3. Now bring your awareness to your toes. Observe any sensations you notice in your toes, such as whether they feel relaxed or tense.

4. Repeat step 3 for the following body parts: your calves, knees, upper legs, lower back, stomach, chest, shoulders, arms, neck, face, then head.

5. As you move through each of the body parts, simply invite yourself to track sensation, so that you are developing your ability to identify the different sensations in your body.

Imagine that you could hop into a special spaceship and zoom up above the river of your life. Imagine that the first stepping-stone you see in the river is your birth, and the stones move all along the river up until the moment of now. From as far a distance as you want, notice five to ten stepping-stones where you experienced a feeling of being under some kind of threat or danger. Take a moment to list these stepping-stones and any associated sensations you notice in your body. This could be something minor, like a bad fall you recovered from, or something more major, like growing up with a violent or unpredictable parent.

Get into your spaceship again and fly back up above the river of your life. Starting from the stepping-stone of your birth, notice all the moments in your life where you felt relaxed, peaceful, and at ease. Notice the corresponding sensations in your body. Notice details about the images of these special moments. Take some time to describe what imagery you observe and any sensations you notice in your body.

_____

_____

_____

_____

_____

_____

_____

_____

_____

_____

_____

_____

_____

_____

_____

_____

_____

_____

_____

PROGRESSIVE MUSCLE RELAXATION

In this relaxation practice, you will focus on slowly tensing and relaxing each muscle group. This practice will develop your ability to focus on different muscle groups and help you become more aware of physical sensations. If you like, you can explore allowing the release of muscular tension on your exhalations.

1. Find a comfortable position seated or lying down.

2. Clench your hands and focus your mind on what the physical sensation of tension is in this part of your body. Which muscles are activated? What does the activation feel like? After you have tensed for a few moments, release.

3. Focus your mind on the physical sensations of relaxation.

4. Proceed to other parts of the body. Squeeze your face muscles and relax. Then separately tense and relax your shoulders, biceps, chest, legs, feet, and toes.

5. You may want to repeat each body part a few times, or you can move directly from one body part to the next.

BREATHING FOCUS

Belly breathing, or abdominal breathing, can be a simple and powerful practice to develop your awareness of the sensations of tension and relaxation.

1. Find a comfortable position seated or lying down.

2. Begin by placing your hands on your lower abdomen so that your palms are resting on the outside of your stomach, toward your hips, and your fingers are splayed open, inward, facing your belly button. If you'd prefer to let your hands rest in your lap, or to place your hands on some other body part that feels more comfortable, feel free to do so. The invitation is to explore mindful breathing, and you may do so in whatever way feels best to you.

3. As you inhale, bring your awareness to the rise of your hands and the expansion of your belly. Think of the incoming breath as an intentional way of bringing in nourishment and support.

4. As you exhale, notice the release of your abdomen and any softening you notice in your belly, back, or pelvis. Think of the outgoing breath as letting go of anything you don't want inside.

5. Feel free to close your eyes at any point if that feels comfortable, and continue to let your awareness focus on the feeling of the rise and fall of your hands and belly. Notice any other feelings of tension or expansion and any feelings of relaxation.

6. Continue this practice for two to five minutes and then rest. If you feel agitated, feel free to take breaks, move your body, and shake your limbs to release excess energy if that feels right for you. As you build greater relaxation and ease, allow yourself to extend your breathing practice each week by a minute or two.

As you begin to explore your relationship to your body, you may discover that finding words to describe what you are sensing is tricky. That's absolutely normal!

Below you will find some universal language that is often used to describe physical sensation. Review the words and then select any that describe your experience when you are feeling tension and when you are feeling relaxation. Write those words in the relevant columns. Feel free to add any words of your own as well.

Descriptive words	When I am relaxed, my body feels . . .	When I am tense, my body feels . . .
Temperature: cold, cool, warm, hot, wet, icy, frozen, burning, chills, like a spark, like a fire, like ice		
Pressure: Pulsing, crushed, cut off, supported, unsupported, still, light, tight, loose, grief		
Air quality: cool, warm, light, directional (from the right, left, above, below), like a feather, like a gust, rushing, stimulating		
Constriction: solid, dense, hot, cold, constricting		
Pain: stabbing, sharp, dagger, hot, cold, ache, twinge		
Tingling: vibrating, numb, tickle, pricking		
Itching: mild, subtle, angry, annoying		
Size: small, large		
Shape: line, circle, flat, like a stone, like a jagged rock		
Absence: nothing, blank, empty		

MELTING TENSION

Working with images that support muscle relaxation is an effective way to develop your capacity to notice contrasting sensations of tension and relaxation. The more you are able to identify muscular relaxation, the more you will build your capacity for parasympathetic tone. If you notice your mind has drifted during the following practice, simply notice that you've drifted, then bring your awareness back to your breath or back to the feeling of relaxation in your body. Imagine that gravity is offering you a gentle invitation to relax and let go a little more.

1. Lie down on your back on a comfortable piece of furniture or, if you prefer, on the floor. Rest your arms alongside your body.

2. Take a moment to focus on your breath. As you focus on your breath, continue to notice if anything else slows or relaxes inside your body.

3. You might imagine that you are a "lazy" animal, such as a dog in front of a fire or a lion in the sun in a field of golden grass. If you notice any sensations of relaxation or softening, take a few moments to live inside that sensation.

4. Invite your body to melt onto the surface that you are lying on. Keep tracking any contrasting sensations of tension and relaxation. Any time you notice sensations of tension, say to yourself, "It's safe to relax."

5. Do this for five to ten minutes and then rest.

One of the main ways that all human beings experience sensations in the body is in relationship to expansion (relaxation) and contraction (tension). The more you practice finding language and images that describe your somatic experience, the more you support your ability to sense what you are feeling. Bring your awareness to your body right now. Notice someplace in your body that feels relaxed. It might be as large an area as your pelvis, or it might be just your little toe. If you aren't able to find someplace inside your body that feels relaxed, allow yourself to remember a time when you felt relaxed. Once you find awareness, answer the following questions.

1. In what body parts do you notice relaxation?

   _____

   _____

   _____

   _____

2. Describe the sensation that accompanies the feeling of relaxation in your body. Does it feel soft, pleasant, settled, open, melting, loose, warm, cool, like a feather, like water, like air, or otherwise?

   _____

   _____

   _____

   _____

3. When you think of relaxation, what image comes to mind? *(Examples: A white, open oval; a bird soaring on the breeze; warm sun; a puppy napping.)*

   _____

   _____

   _____

   _____

CALMING BEACH AND OCEAN RHYTHM BREATHING

In the following practice, you can explore forming mental images or pictures to support feelings of relaxation and calm. Feel free to incorporate as many senses as you'd like, including smell, sight, touch, and sound. As you explore your beach image, include the smell of the ocean salt or the feeling of a warm breeze touching your skin.

1. Find a comfortable spot, either sitting or lying down.

2. Loosen any tight clothing, such as a waistband or belt, and begin to allow your awareness to settle on your breathing. Imagine yourself on a warm, calm beach. You might imagine that your fingers are moving through the warm, soft sand. You might hear the sound of seagulls or children's laughter in the distance.

3. Bring your awareness to the sound of the ocean gently lapping on the shore. You might notice the slight increase in volume as the waves roll onto the shore and then the subtle decrease in volume as the water moves back out to the sea.

4. As you continue to imagine and sense the sounds of the ocean, notice the gentle rise and fall of your breath.

5. Do this for five to ten minutes and then rest.

When you carry too much tension in your body, you use up valuable energy, and over time, tension can create discomfort and pain. Relieving tension requires enhancing your awareness of the contrasting sensations of relaxation and deepening your moment-to-moment awareness of the sensations in your body.

Turn your awareness inside your body and notice how your body feels right now. Notice someplace in your body that feels tense or tight. If you aren't able to find someplace inside your body that feels contracted, try squeezing your hand for a few seconds and noticing the sensations. Once you find awareness, answer the following questions.

1. In what body parts do you notice contraction and tension?

_____

_____

_____

_____

2. Describe the sensation that accompanies the feeling of tension in your body. Does it feel tight, squeezed, hard, firm, uncomfortable, unpleasant, tiring, like a rock, like a ball, or otherwise?

_____

_____

_____

_____

3. When you think of tension, what image comes to mind? *(Examples: A black ball; a spiky gray rock; a dark circle; a sad face.)*

_____

_____

_____

_____

Key Takeaways

Becoming aware of tension and learning how to relax your body are important for your overall health and well-being. Chronic stress and physical tension have been referred to as silent killers, as they compromise the immune system and can have a serious impact on your day-to-day mood and functioning.

- Physical tension is increasingly recognized by the scientific and medical community as a major contributor to persistent and chronic disease, such as heart disease, cancer, gastrointestinal problems, and sleep disorders.

- Notice the kinds of experiences that create tension in your body and the kinds of experiences that support feelings of relaxation.

- Practice finding language that describes the sensations you experience in your body.

- Notice when you are experiencing sensations of tension in your body.

- Support your ability to relax by bringing your awareness to the tension and using breath, progressive relaxation, or images to begin changing your responses to stress.

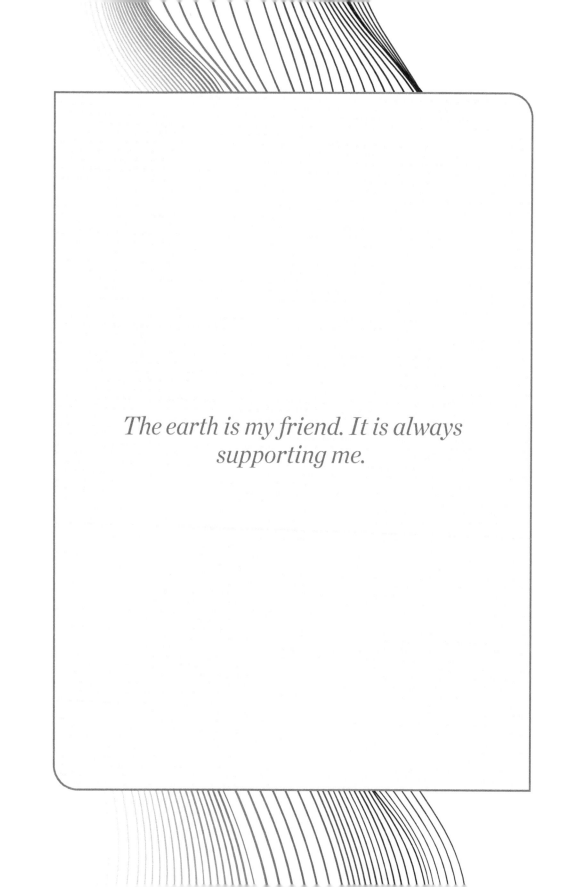

The earth is my friend. It is always supporting me.

CHAPTER FOUR

Embodying the Moment with Grounding Techniques

In life, you have circumstances that feel heavy, and you may notice resulting tension, stress, or confusion. You may also have been carrying this heaviness around for much of your life, and over time, you may begin to feel that there isn't much support for the weight you are carrying.

It is also likely that the different roles you play and the directions in which you are being pulled will leave you feeling overwhelmed, overstimulated, overtired, and disconnected from yourself. When this happens, it is important that you are able to notice these feelings and bring yourself back to your body and back into the present moment.

Grounding techniques often use the available senses—sound, touch, smell, taste, and sight—to immediately connect you with the here and now, including "grounding" your feet to the earth below. It is a reliable way to support your nervous system and move into a state of rest and digest. When you practice grounding, you are developing your ability to shift your mood and experience consciously and intentionally.

Putting Grounding Techniques into Practice

Grounding is a powerful tool for healing trauma because your ability to direct your awareness to the ground supports relaxation, which generally reduces states of activation. Often, simply by directing your attention to the floor or the back of your chair or letting your gaze rest on something soothing, you can quickly reduce sympathetic states in which you feel distress and bring yourself back into a parasympathetic regulation in which you you feel more at ease.

Grounding can be likened to ice melting. You might think of your focused attention like the warmth of the sun, and as you direct your awareness toward parasympathetic sensations of relaxation, support, or pleasant feelings of the weight of your body resting, you are melting sympathetic activation from your body.

In the following chapter you'll be introduced to a variety of ways in which you can begin to practice grounding in your day-to-day life. The fundamental concepts that you want to explore in your grounding practice are:

1. The somatic sensations of physical relaxation.

2. The somatic sensations that arise out of bringing your awareness to the contact of your body with physical support, such as your chair or the floor.

3. The somatic sensations that arise as you allow your available senses to orient you to the physical and sensory experience of your immediate environment.

4. The somatic sensations that arise as you bring your awareness to the solidity and stability of the floor, a chair, objects in your immediate environment, or the awareness of boundaries.

When you support yourself by self-directing your awareness, your body is better able to receive messages about support, location, solidity, and boundaries, and it can begin to move naturally into relief and relaxation.

Think about a time or a situation when you felt connected to the earth. This might have been a time when you were out in your backyard on a sunny day with your shoes off and the sun on your face. Maybe you felt connected to the earth while you were planting flowers in your garden or sitting on a rock at the summit of a hike. Write about the memory and make note of any physical sensation, emotion, or awareness that arises.

_____

_____

_____

_____

_____

_____

_____

_____

_____

_____

_____

_____

_____

_____

_____

_____

_____

_____

_____

Another way to ground yourself in the present moment and feel more embodied is through imagery. This practice makes use of an image connected to a state of being that supports your capacity to feel at ease. Reflect on a time in the last twenty-four hours, week, or month when you felt most like yourself—a moment of feeling at ease, present, neutral, or content. As you connect with this experience, notice the image or memory that comes to mind. What senses can you tap into in your imagination? Write down what you are seeing and how your body reacts.

_____

_____

_____

_____

_____

_____

_____

_____

Next, write about what you are feeling in your body as you tune in to the image or memory in your mind. What sensations are you aware of? Where do you feel them in your body?

_____

_____

_____

_____

_____

_____

_____

_____

Spiritual teacher and writer Eckhart Tolle says, "The moment you realize you are not present, you are present." Even if you are experiencing dysregulation or discomfort in your body, as you begin to tune in to what those sensations are, you create more awareness, which creates more space, which can create more ground, which creates more stabilization. Right now, ask yourself with a spirit of curiosity, as though you were a trusted friend, "How does my body feel in this moment?" Spend some time to describe what you are feeling in as much detail as possible.

MAKING CONTACT WITH THE FLOOR

One way that you can establish or deepen somatic grounding at any moment is by directing your awareness away from the external environment to your feet making contact with the floor. Find a seated position and move your feet forward and backward along the floor. Then move them side to side along the floor until your feet feel a bit more connected to the floor. Now feel your pelvis, back, and buttocks being supported by the chair. Notice that the floor extends through the entire room, that the floor goes underneath the walls and connects this room with other rooms, that the building you are in is supported by the earth, and that the earth beneath you is part of the fabric of the entire planet. Write about where in your body you are experiencing sensations of comfort or support, as well as reflections about how extensive the support of the ground is underneath you at any moment.

THE CROWN TECHNIQUE

The crown technique helps focus your mind on the feeling between you and the earth. It is a simple grounding practice that is effective at bringing awareness into your body and the present moment. You might like to try this practice with bare feet to offer more sensations to your body.

1. Find a comfortable seat in a chair.

2. Rest one hand on top of your head. Allow your grip to be firm but not hard.

3. Close your eyes if you'd like, or keep them open with a soft gaze. Notice how your hand feels on your head and notice the weight of your hand.

4. Notice if you become more aware of your feet on the ground as your hand rests on your head.

5. See if you can hold your awareness of both the feeling of your feet on the ground and the feeling of your hand on your head at the same time. Do this for a few minutes and then rest.

GROUNDING THROUGH THE EARTH

All grounding techniques focus on connecting your body to the earth. Your body has an electrical conductivity to the earth, and if you increase your skin-to-earth contact, the earth acts as a large battery that can balance, recharge, and ground your body.

1. Try walking barefoot on the carpet of your home and notice the sensations you feel.

2. Try walking barefoot on the linoleum or tile in your bathroom, kitchen, or elsewhere and notice the sensations you feel.

3. Try walking barefoot on the grass.

4. Try placing your hands on firm ground and loose soil and notice what you feel in your body.

5. Try wrapping your arms around the trunk of a tree. Notice what you feel in your body. It may feel strange to do, but it's amazing how powerful it can be to connect with nature like this.

Orienting is a foundational somatic therapy practice in healing unresolved trauma. The capacity to orient to one's environment has two different modes: exploratory and defensive.

Defensive orientation is what occurs when you feel under threat, and exploratory orientation is what happens when you feel safe. Exploratory orientation involves allowing the head and neck to move freely and the eyes to take in whatever there is to see in the immediate environment. This movement of the head and neck can reduce tension around the first and second cervical vertebrae and increase blood flow to your vertebral artery, which supplies blood to the brain stem and vagus nerve. The vagus nerve influences your heart rate and breathing and is involved in how you perceive, react to, and recover from stress. When the vagus nerve is activated, you operate through a system that Dr. Stephen Porges refers to as the "social engagement system." When you are in this state, you feel a playful mixture of activation and calm that allows you to feel safe and alert.

It is important to restore exploratory orientation, as it supports your capacity for curiosity, sensory input, self-regulation, grounding, and mindfulness.

1. First, look down right in front of your body. Write about what you see.

    _____

    _____

2. Look ten feet in front of you, or if you are in a room, look across the room to the farthest wall. Describe what you see at this distance.

    _____

    _____

3. Now look into the distance. If you are in a room, look out a window and notice something as far off in the distance as you can. Write down what you see.

    _____

    _____

4. Finish by observing how you feel after doing this practice. Do you feel more in your body, more present, more relaxed, or otherwise?

    _____

    _____

GROUNDING THROUGH WATER

Around 60 percent of your body is made up of water. Water is the base for all the fluids in your body, and all of your feelings, thoughts, and actions are a result of your body's chemical or electrical impulses passing through water. Therefore, the color, image, and movement of water is a wonderful resource that can be a reminder of your natural human capacity as fresh, flowing, changing, and resilient. Because of this, water can be used to ground in the same way the physical earth is used for grounding.

Select one or more of the following water experiences to try grounding through water for yourself.

- Let warm water run over your hands and arms in the sink. Notice how the temperature feels. Rub a fragrant soap or lotion into your hands and breathe in the smell. Bring your attention to the feelings of your fingers and hands moving on each other.

- Take a shower and allow yourself to spend time just focusing on the sensations of the warm water on your body.

- Run a warm bath and allow yourself to feel the boundaries of the bathtub as you float in the water. Feel free to add your favorite bubble bath or bath salts to enhance your sensory experience.

Bringing awareness to the back of your body is another useful grounding technique.

1. Begin by finding a comfortable position in which your body feels both relaxed and alert.

2. Start at your feet and notice the feeling of contact starting at the bottom of your body, and then track any places where your body is making contact with the chair and back support. Let your body relax and soften into the support of the chair.

3. Notice places where you feel a lot of contact, or notice that your body is releasing to accept the support of the chair, and notice where there are lighter places of contact.

4. Notice the alignment of your spine. Are there places where you are hunched forward?

5. Are there places where you are leaning too far back?

When you are finished, look at the illustration and place circles where you were aware of sensations of contact with the chair. Annotate the illustration, using words or drawings, for any other sensations you felt in your body. Notice places in the body where you feel pleasant or unpleasant sensations.

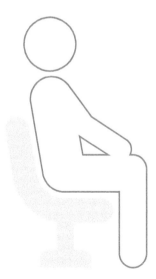

GROUNDING YOGA POSE

Yoga is inherently a grounding form of movement. In yoga, "ground" serves as an adjective to describe a "centered, grounded feeling" and as a verb to mean "to physically ground down." One of the basic tenets of yoga is that each posture contains oppositional direction: movement toward the earth and toward the sky. In every yoga posture, you are bringing mindful attention to actively take support from the ground in order to support the natural alignment in the body. The following instructions will guide you into "child's pose." It is a restorative body posture that lowers your head beneath your heart, signaling to the nervous system that it's time to slow down.

1. Find an open space on the floor. Feel free to use a carpet, blanket, or yoga mat for added comfort.

2. Come down to the floor on your hands and knees in a tabletop position.

3. From the tabletop position, spread your knees out as wide as is comfortable, guiding your hips over your heels and pulling your big toes together to touch.

4. Now, slowly walk your palms forward and allow your hands to be spread out across the floor. Let your forehead gently rest on the floor.

5. Allow your belly to relax. With each exhalation, imagine that gravity is inviting you to release more and more. Allow your body to melt into the floor.

6. Do this practice for five to ten minutes.

Tracking how you feel throughout the week can help you begin to have more awareness about the changing states of your body and the different stimuli that are a part of your changing states. As you increase awareness about what feels pleasurable and grounding, you will have more control over how to bring your body back into regulated states in moments of stress or overwhelm.

Use the following chart during the coming week to deepen your somatic awareness about moments when you feel most grounded and at ease. You can fill it out in the moment if you have this book handy or return to the book later in the day to reflect on your memories of feeling grounded.

Day/ Time	Surroundings	Occurrence	Sensations	Where I Feel
Saturday morning	In my living room in my favorite chair. The light is soft, and the room is quiet.	I am reading a book.	Relaxed and warm.	In my chest, pelvis, and feet.

Focusing on the five senses is a wonderful way to ground yourself. Working backward from 5, use your senses to list things around you that you can sense. If you do not have access to five senses, you can do this exercise focusing on the senses that are available to you and add additional elements on those senses. Write about what you notice.

5 Things You Can Hear

Turn your attention to your sense of sound. Experiment with noticing sounds that are close to you and sounds that are farther away. Write down five things you can hear.

_____

_____

_____

_____

_____

4 Things You Can See

List four things that you can see. You might choose to experiment with distance by first seeing things that are close to you and then moving your gaze farther away.

_____

_____

_____

_____

3 Things You Can Touch

Notice three things you can touch and feel and write them down.

_____

_____

_____

2 Things You Can Smell

Notice and write down two things you can smell.

_____

_____

1 Thing You Can Taste

What does the inside of your mouth taste like—coffee, toothpaste, or even nothing? Describe it here.

_____

ANCHORING PHRASE OR AFFIRMATION

Your inner dialogue is a crucial aspect of psychological health. The way you speak to yourself has a significant impact on how you feel and who you believe yourself to be. Therefore, being intentional about the supportive language you offer yourself can be an anchor for feeling grounded and safe in your body. You might choose to offer yourself grounding phrases at specific times of the day, or affirmations might be supports that you can reach for during moments of anxiety or frustration.

Below are some grounding affirmations for you to choose from. Take some time to say each of these out loud to yourself. Repeat each one three times. When you are finished, you might like to write down any that resonated with you on a sticky note and place it somewhere prominent in your home or write it down as a note in your phone so that you can refer back to it during your daily life.

- I center myself with the ease of my breath.

- I am supported and protected.

- I am supported by the ground beneath my feat.

- I am safe in my body.

- I am exactly where I am meant to be.

- Even when life feels fast, I can slow down.

- I have space, and I can take as much time as I need.

Key Takeaways

When you are noticing stress or physical tension in your body, grounding is a reliable way to feel supported by the ground in order to move into a state of rest. When you practice grounding, you are developing your ability to shift your mood and experience from something that is unpleasant to something pleasant. Grounding can also help you come out of states of overwhelm or exhaustion into a state of rest and clarity. Some grounding practices include the following:

- Connecting with the felt sensations of your feet making contact with the floor beneath you.

- Connecting with the felt sensations of your body touching the chair beneath you.

- Connecting with the grounding sensations or images of water on your body.

- Using your senses to come into the present moment and into your body.

- Using your eyes to orient yourself to the space around you and to explore what you see up close and at a far distance.

- Connecting with images where you feel most like yourself.

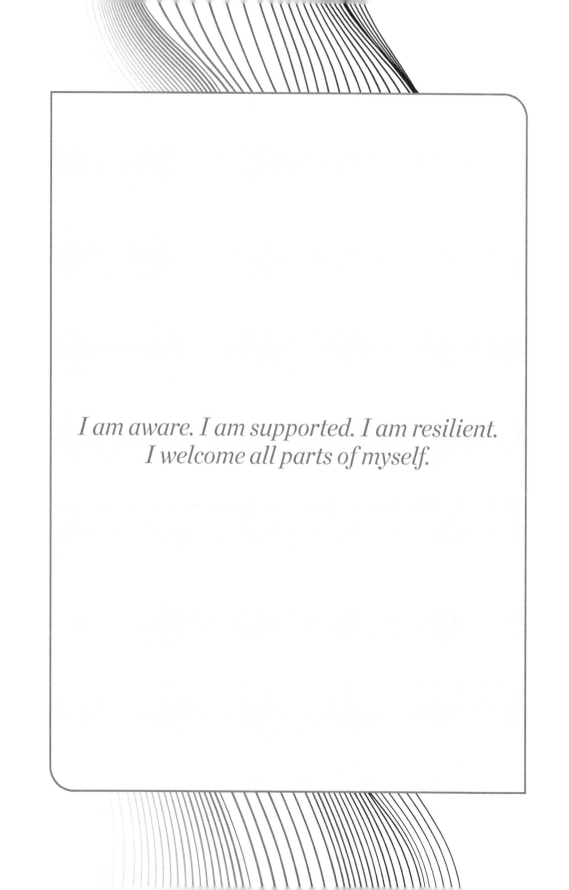

I am aware. I am supported. I am resilient. I welcome all parts of myself.

CHAPTER FIVE

Safely Revisiting Memories with Pendulation Techniques

Pendulation is a somatic therapy tool that can help you cope with the distress and discomfort that may arise when healing from trauma. In the same way that a pendulum moves back and forth between opposite ends, you, too, are capable of moving between states of activation and states of calm. The goal of pendulation work is to strengthen this natural rhythm in your nervous system so that you may more easily shift from a state of sympathetic arousal (alertness and action) to a place of parasympathetic engagement (rest and calm).

In addition to restoring resilience and flexibility to the nervous system, other benefits of pendulation include an increased capacity to observe different emotional states, a greater ability to self-soothe, and an increased tolerance of situations or sensations that are ambiguous or complex and may be difficult to easily make sense of.

Putting Pendulation into Practice

For those healing from trauma, either revising traumatic memories or simply tuning in to unpleasant sensations can result in sympathetic arousal, such as a quickening heartbeat or feelings of numbness. Through the pendulation activities in this chapter, you will learn to take a moment to feel and notice these responses and then scan your body to find a place that feels calm and relaxed so that you can shift your awareness there.

It is crucial that you cultivate a feeling of safety in your nervous system before revisiting traumatic memory, because it is your ability to feel safe in the present that is an essential aspect of processing traumatic memory. The capacity to feel safe allows your mind-body connection to begin to process that the threat you experienced is in the past and you are no longer in danger.

Pendulation is one of the main methods used in somatic therapy to guide the nervous system toward increased balance, as well as to expand your ability to notice the positive aspects of your experience so you are not solely focused on the negative. This expansion of noticing positive aspects of your experience alongside the negative widens your window of tolerance to accept more of the variety of fluctuations in state and emotion that you inevitably encounter in life.

Many natural cycles on earth are defined by the movements of expansion and contraction. Think about how the wings of birds move, or the rising and falling of waves. Indeed, your own path in life does not follow a linear trajectory. Where have you observed the rhythm of pendulation in nature, your own life, or the lives of others?

_____

_____

_____

_____

_____

_____

_____

_____

_____

_____

_____

_____

_____

_____

_____

_____

_____

_____

_____

_____

Take some time to reflect on what kinds of stimuli activate a sympathetic response in your nervous system. You might notice a spike in adrenaline, more rapid breathing, tightness in your musculature, an increased heart rate, constriction in your chest, or feelings of anxiety or fear. Write about what changes you notice in your body, as well as identifying what kinds of environments, situations, behaviors, or events trigger a sympathetic response.

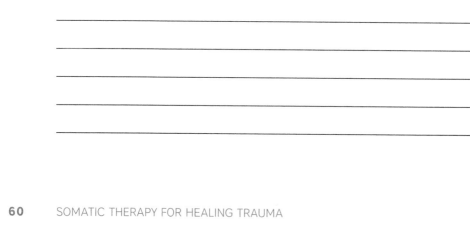

As you continue to make your way through this workbook, there are times when you will be called upon to reflect on memories about difficult experiences you may have had. The goal is to bring to mind memories that activate a mild emotional and physical response rather than recollections of events that cause you to feel distressed or overwhelmed.

It will help to imagine your response on a scale of 1 to 10, with 1 being a faint response and 10 being overwhelming. Your activation should fall only within the range of 2 to 4.

1 ——— 2 ——— 3 ——— 4 ——— 5 ——— 6 ——— 7 ——— 8 ——— 9 ——— 10

Calm   *Lightly activated*   *Moderately*   *Distressed*   *Overwhelmed*
                                    activated

While the content of such a memory will be unique for each person, here are a few examples that might help put you in the ballpark of what it could be:

- An encounter with an unfriendly neighbor on the street or in the elevator.

- Something your partner or friend did that caused a spike in irritation or concern.

- Thinking of an important meeting with a big new client at work.

Once you have brought some to mind, write down a short, simple phrase or headline that describes five different memories that fall within the appropriate activation range.

1. _____

2. _____

3. _____

4. _____

5. _____

When you encounter an activity in the rest of the book that asks you to call upon a memory within the lower range of activation, you can use the examples you have written here. If possible, conduct such activities with the assistance of a therapist. If you do not have a therapist with you and feel overwhelmed, try a grounding or safe space exercise from the book that helps bring you back into a regulated state.

In somatic therapy, a resource is anything that brings sensations of relaxation, safety, comfort, and support to your system. Use the space provided to describe a resource in your life. It could be a beloved friend, pet, imaginary figure, or fictional character. It may even be an object, such as a weighted blanket, or something you do, such as taking a break outside in nature. How has this resource been helpful in the past? When you bring it to mind, what sensations do you observe?

Take a moment to bring to mind the image of the resource you wrote about in the previous prompt and observe the sensations in your body. You could choose a low-level stimulus from the activation reflection on page 61—something that would be a 2 to 4 on a scale of 1 to 10. Imagine that you were just lightly touching the memory with your hand, then come back to the image of your resource. What did you notice as you moved between the activating memory and the resource? Describe any shift in your thoughts, emotions, or bodily sensations with as much detail as possible.

_____

_____

_____

_____

_____

_____

_____

_____

_____

_____

_____

_____

_____

_____

_____

_____

_____

_____

_____

PENDULATING WITH THE EYES

In early developmental moments, babies intuitively know how to take in as much stimulus as their systems can handle and then look away to reorganize, orient, and integrate. Somatic therapy encourages you to apply this same principle to regulating your nervous system. When you learn to switch between stimulation and rest, you can achieve a more sustainable balance.

Opening and closing your eyes is a helpful way to track sensations of activation and sensations of grounding or settling. This simple practice invites you to become more familiar with the pendulation between activation and settling by opening and closing your eyes and noticing what feelings and sensations emerge.

1. Allow your eyes to close for a few moments and wait until you feel some sensations of settling and grounding. Notice the sensations of settling and where in your body you feel this.

2. Then let your eyes open and notice if there are any sensations of activation inside your body. The aim is to refine your ability to sense activating sensations, even if these are subtle and pleasant.

3. Try slowly opening and closing your eyes a few times and tracking any changes of sensation inside your body.

4. Allow your eyes to guide you where they want to look. Depending on where your gaze rests, continue to notice whether there are sensations of sympathetic activation or parasympathetic regulation.

Using language to describe sensations and emotions that you feel in your body has been proven to ease states of arousal. However, finding words that accurately describe somatic sensation is a little bit like learning a new language, and it can take time to find words that match what you are feeling in your body. The following exercise will help you begin to develop a vocabulary for sensation to enhance your somatic awareness and support pendulation.

Take a moment to think about the last time you felt peaceful and at ease, then answer the following questions. There are some word options to choose from for each question; however, you can simply use them as inspiration to help you think up your own words if you wish. You can also use the list of words in chapter 3 (page 32) if you need to.

1. What I'm feeling in my body is (*Example*: *calm, stable, peaceful, whole, full, light, warm, solid, clear*):

   _____

   _____

   _____

   _____

   _____

   _____

2. The image I have in my mind is (*Example*: *a green forest, a calm lake, the color blue, a circle, a tall glass of water*):

   _____

   _____

   _____

   _____

   _____

   _____

continued > > >

3. The gesture or movement that my body wants to make right now is (*Example*: *to open my arms wide, to close my eyes, to spin around, to lie down, to bring my hands to my face, to dance, to shake, to wiggle*):

_____

_____

_____

_____

_____

_____

_____

_____

4. After this exercise, what I'm noticing in my body is (*Example*: *calm, stable, peaceful, whole, full, light, warm, solid, clear*):

_____

_____

_____

_____

_____

_____

_____

_____

PENDULATION WITH MOVEMENT

Your body is always in motion; however, there is a difference between moving without awareness and bringing mindful attention to the sensations of your movement. In this practice, you will experience pendulation in action by mindfully opening and closing your body posture. In doing this, you will support your abilities to notice feelings of activation and self-direct toward regulation. This creates a foundation for being able to self-soothe and self-regulate in moments of discomfort or distress.

1. Cross your arms over your chest, as if you're giving yourself a hug. Let your head bow down to your chest. Notice the sensations of this posture. Notice where your gaze wants to go. Notice whether your eyes want to stay open or closed. Notice your breath. Notice your legs and feet.

2. Now sense into your body for an impulse to open your posture. Move very slowly so that you can feel every micro-sensation of this movement. Allow yourself to begin to uncurl. Notice your head begin to lift. Notice your spine lengthening. Notice how your arms want to move as your body opens. Notice your breath. Notice your face muscles. Notice your legs and feet.

3. Continue this movement a few more times. Move in slow motion, slower than you may have ever moved, and stay fully present in the experience of the movement. Notice any sensations, images, and associated emotions that come along with the movement.

As you develop your capacity for somatic sensation, you will likely become more aware when you experience unpleasant sensations of fear, anxiety, fatigue, stress, or sadness. This is a normal part of the process, and in time, you will begin bringing ease to yourself more quickly.

When you witness an emotion or sensation that is uncomfortable, you make more space for the feeling, which means you are able to listen to the information the feeling may be offering to you. Working with images is a supportive element of somatic therapy, and developing this practice is a great way to tap into your creative capacities. This exercise also aims to expand your window of tolerance, demonstrating to your body-mind your increasing capacity to be with both positive and negative feelings at once and develop your feeling of safety.

1. Allow yourself to think about a recent memory or event that caused some uncomfortable turbulence in your body. Notice where you are experiencing the sensation; picture what it looks like; notice its shape, movement, or quality; or imagine the feeling as an object.

2. Now imagine the opposite of this image. Picture an image that is pleasant, soothing, and grounding. This might be a place where you love to sit and feel relaxed, cozy, and safe, or maybe it's a beautiful tree, swaying gently in the breeze atop a quiet hill.

3. Draw your images in the boxes provided.

4. When you have finished drawing these, take your time to pendulate back and forth by looking at the activating image and then allowing your gaze to take time to rest on the opposite image.

5. As you pendulate between the two images, your aim is to track your body's gradual diminishment of sympathetic activation toward expanding sensations of parasympathetic engagement. Allow yourself to spend so much time with the opposite image that you start to feel sensations of ease, support, groundedness, softening in muscle tone, and deepening of your breath.

Activating Image

Opposite Image

PENDULATING BETWEEN THINKING AND SENSING

Has your mind ever felt stuck in a loop of negative thoughts that you can't seem to stop? The following somatic practice demonstrates how to pendulate from your thinking to sensing inside your body. This can break the cycle of negative thinking and allow you to tap into your felt experience in the present moment. Try this practice when you notice you are caught in thinking.

1. Notice a repeated thought you are experiencing.

2. Accept the thought pattern with compassion and non-judgment. Say, "Hello, repeated thought. I am aware of you, and you are welcome here."

3. Now bring awareness to your body. Sense into someplace inside that feels at ease. Notice your breath moving through your body or the feeling of the air on your skin.

4. If the thought pulls you back, simply notice it and bring your attention back to your body.

5. Continue to pendulate between any thoughts that arise and bringing your awareness back to sensing your body.

6. See if you can hang out with the feelings in your body a little longer each time you do this practice.

7. Notice any shifts in your experience. Notice any spaciousness, easing, or slowing down that occur in your thought rhythm.

You can't always know what kind of stimulation will cause disruption to your nervous system or what that disruption will feel like when it occurs. However, you can begin to build a map that deepens your self-awareness about what kind of stimuli tend to change your state of being and how you can bring yourself back into greater balance.

If you have certain traumatic memories from your life that you would like to work on, you can use the following map to begin making note of those experiences. Select two to five words to describe the event, as if you were writing a newspaper headline.

Once you have your title in mind, write it down in the space provided and then describe where you feel it in your body, along with any description or imagery of the sensation. After this, note where in the body feels the opposite (i.e., calm and safe) and how you would describe it. Space is provided to do this for two different memories. Feel free to use the list of words in chapter 3 on page 32 to describe your sensations.

	Example	My Memory Sensations 1	My Memory Sensations 2
Short title or phrase for the activating memory	*Falling down the basement steps.*		
Where I feel activated in my body	*Upper chest and throat.*		
Description or imagery for the sensations	*Spiky and tight.*		
Place in the body that feels the opposite (calm and safe)	*My pelvis and butt.*		
Description or imagery of pleasant sensations	*Solid and quiet. Like a circle.*		

The following exercise will support pendulation and help you widen your window of tolerance.

1. Find a comfortable seated position and take a few moments to attend to feelings of groundedness in your body. Think of a recent moment when you experienced irritation or reactivity.

2. Tune into your felt-sense of your body. Notice whatever images and emotions are associated with your experience.

3. Shift your awareness to the back of your body. Allow your entire sense of self to rest in the support and contact with the chair. Notice the contact of your feet on the ground. Take a moment to look around your space and let your eyes rest wherever they want.

4. Allow your awareness to return to the irritating stimulus and notice if there are any changes in your sensations and experience. Notice any details that you might not have noticed before.

5. Return to the sensations at the back of your body.

6. Try holding your awareness on both the activating sensations and the resourced sensations at the same time.

When you are finished, reflect on the different sensations you experienced by answering these questions.

In step 2, what unpleasant activating sensations did you notice?

_____

_____

What message do you think these sensations were telling you?

_____

_____

In step 3, what resourced sensations did you notice?

_____

_____

What message do you think these were telling you?

_____

_____

In step 4, did you notice a decrease in activation when you returned to the unpleasant sensation?

_____

_____

Finally, write about what it felt like to hold both the activating and resourced sensations at the same time and how this skill could help you on your healing journey.

_____

_____

_____

_____

_____

_____

_____

_____

_____

RAIN (RECOGNIZE, ALLOW, INVESTIGATE, AND NURTURE)

The RAIN technique is a wonderful practice that supports your ability to notice sympathetic activation and engage in pendulation to down-regulate to a calm parasympathetic state. The meditation teacher Michele McDonald introduced the RAIN practice, and psychologist Tara Brach modified and popularized RAIN as follows.

Take a moment to think of a memory with a low degree of activation. The memory you choose should have an activation range of 2 to 4, on a scale of 1 to 10 (see page 61).

1. Close your eyes for a moment to notice what you are feeling.

2. **Recognize** by asking yourself, "What am I noticing inside my body right now?" Observe what comes up.

3. **Allow** the experience to be here, just as it is. Say to the sensations you are experiencing, "There is space for you to be here." Notice any shifts or changes in your somatic experience.

4. **Investigate** what you are experiencing with gentleness and curiosity.

    a. Where are the sensations strongest in your body?

    b. What is the most difficult or painful thing you are believing?

    c. What is this part needing?

5. **Nurture** yourself with self-compassion. Invite a compassionate part of yourself to be present. Notice where you feel this compassionate part in your body. Allow your awareness to settle on any area of your body that feels the opposite of the sensations of activation.

PENDULATING WITH A LOW-ACTIVATION MEMORY

Choosing a low-activation memory will allow you to focus on the movement of pendulation between sympathetic response and parasympathetic response.

1. Begin by sitting in a comfortable position. You can have your eyes open or closed, whichever feels best to you.

2. Building on the grounding techniques from chapter 4, start to scan your body for any part that feels settled or pleasant. This might be a large area of your body, such as where your pelvis connects with the chair, or it can be a tiny spot, like your pinkie finger.

3. Think of a recent experience that created a little bit of activation. This might be an email you received, an exchange with someone on the street, or an interaction with your partner. The memory you choose should have an activation range of 2 to 4, on a scale of 1 to 10 (see page 61).

4. As you recall the event, focus your awareness on any difficult sensations that arise. If the full feeling of activation is too unpleasant, try taking just a little bit of the sensation.

5. After a few moments of tracking the sensations of activation, return to the place in your body that feels settled or pleasant.

Key Takeaways

Pendulation is the natural rhythm of expansion and contraction that occurs in a resilient and healthy nervous system when you move between states of sympathetic arousal (alertness and action) and parasympathetic engagement (rest and calm).

- Pendulation is an essential aspect of trauma processing, and it will also help you develop the skills to down-regulate your system in moments of dysregulation.

- Pendulation guides the nervous system toward balance and expands your capacity to notice positive aspects of your experience. The ability to notice both the positive and negative aspects of your experience widens your window of tolerance.

- Pendulation helps you fortify resourced states of being in order to build your capacity to tolerate discomfort and be with uncomfortable aspects of your experience with greater ease.

- Developing language for sensation is a key skill that helps you regulate your nervous system.

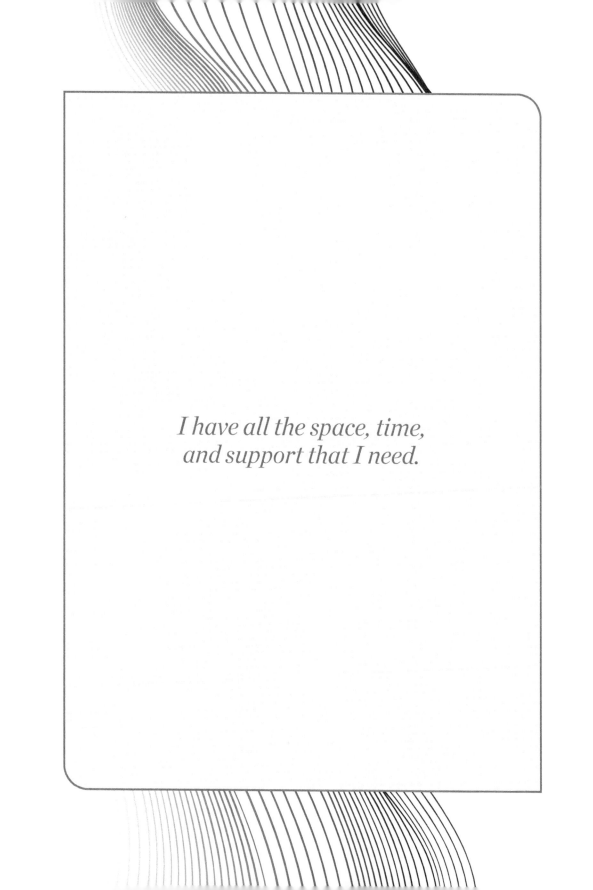

I have all the space, time,
and support that I need.

CHAPTER SIX

Integrating Trauma with Titration Techniques

Trauma is sometimes defined as "too much, too fast, too soon." Therefore, when you are processing trauma, you want to create the opposite condition: just a little bit, very slow, at just the right time.

In chemistry, *titration* refers to safely mixing two substances one drop at a time. Imagine there are two beakers with volatile liquids that would explode if mixed together all at once. Now imagine if you gradually added a tiny drop of one to the other, allowing for a series of minor chemical reactions to take place, so the two liquids can integrate fully to safely produce a new substance that causes no harm.

This same principle applies to processing trauma. Rather than overwhelming your nervous system with the intense sensations that linger from your trauma, you gradually expose your system to these feelings one drop at a time. This allows your nervous system time and space to safely tap into trapped sensations from trauma, reduce their intensity, and integrate them into your experience. In the following chapter you will learn a variety of approaches for titration and how to use it to support processing traumatic memory.

Putting Titration into Practice

Titration allows you to be present with just a little bit of activation at a time, which has the benefit of creating more space and allows for the innate, natural pendulation between parasympathetic and sympathetic activation to become established again. It is powerfully healing to *refuse to leave your experience* and to learn to be present with the original traumatic memory you experienced in a new way.

Since trauma caused your body to experience too much, too soon, you want to be precise in your chemistry about how you moderate revisiting traumatic experiences of the past. Titration is the act of slowing down your response, be it emotional or physiological. You will become the director of pacing your nervous system processing, making it extremely slow, in effect opening up more space for the settling and integration for the activation and arousal responses and associated information.

A common phrase or image used in titration technique is being with "just the edge" of an emotion or sensation. It can be helpful to explore this concept sensorily and somatically. Find a medium-size object, such as a book or a pillow, and hold it out in front of you. Take a moment to look at the entire object. Do you notice that it looks all-encompassing in your field of vision? Now direct your attention to the edges of the object. Do you notice that you can still identify the object but have more space in your field of vision?

Reflect on a sensation or emotion that has been overwhelming for you in the past, such as anxiety, panic, or anger. What has your experience with it been?

_____

_____

_____

_____

_____

_____

Now reflect on how it would feel to safely experience just the edge of the emotion or sensation. How might that feel? How could this help you?

_____

_____

_____

_____

_____

_____

When your nervous system is activated by a trauma response of traumatic memory, you can experience what is referred to as a flooding of overwhelming emotions or sensations. Titration techniques aim to introduce just a drop of a difficult emotion or sensation so that you can make sense of it, process it, and integrate it into your experience without being re-traumatized.

Think of another overwhelming emotion or sensation. In the left-hand column of the following chart, write down words that describe what you would feel if you were flooded by the emotion or sensation. In the right-hand column, write down words that describe what it would feel like to experience just a drop.

Overwhelmed (Flooding)	Titrated (Just a Drop)

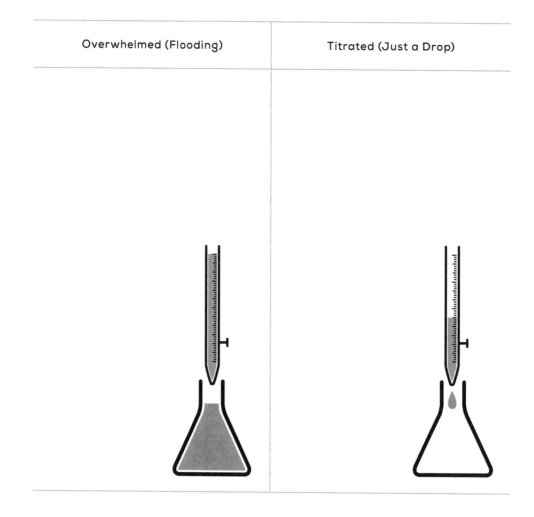

When you are working with a traumatic memory or experience, imagining placing the memory or feeling outside of your body is a way to create more space that supports titration. Take a moment to think of an activating experience, a 2 to 4 on a scale of 1 to 10 (see page 61). Take a moment to notice and record the sensations in your body.

_____

_____

_____

_____

_____

_____

_____

Now imagine placing the feeling or memory out across the room, out the window, or down the block. How much distance did your imagination offer in order to feel some relief in your body? What shift in psychical sensations did you notice in your body? What change in emotion did you feel?

_____

_____

_____

_____

_____

_____

_____

When you experience physiological arousal, you may feel that the experience is too overwhelming for your body to hold. Therefore, in trauma reprocessing, you can draw on your imaginative and creative capacities to work with size as another way to titrate. Take a moment to think of an activating experience, a 2 to 4 on a scale of 1 to 10 (page 61). Now imagine that you can shrink the experience down. For instance, you might imagine the event as if it were just a few inches tall, like the size of a toy truck. Draw or write about your image in the space provided.

The window of tolerance is a wonderful tool to track when you are grounded and resourced and when you are feeling dysregulated. It is composed of three main zones:

- **Hyperarousal**, or the fight-or-flight response, is often characterized by hyper-vigilance, anxiety, fear, and racing thoughts.

- **Hypoarousal**, or the freeze response, may cause feelings of emotional numbness, dissociation, emptiness, or paralysis.

- **Optimum arousal** is the preferred zone to heal stress and trauma symptoms. In this zone, you are oriented to the here and now, have access to your full cognitive and physical capacities, can think creatively, can be reasonable and rational, have compassion for yourself, and have empathy for others.

Window of Tolerance

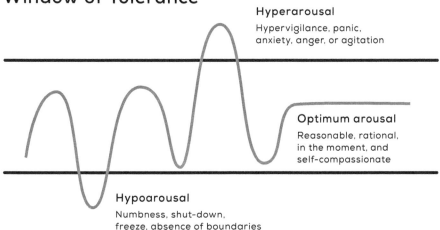

Hyperarousal
Hypervigilance, panic, anxiety, anger, or agitation

Optimum arousal
Reasonable, rational, in the moment, and self-compassionate

Hypoarousal
Numbness, shut-down, freeze, absence of boundaries

Complete the statements on the following pages to build your awareness of what each state is like for you. This will help you recognize the different features of each state and support your ability to be aware of your different states and move into the optimal arousal zone during times of dysregulation.

Hyperarousal

1. The types of experiences, feelings, people, or environments that can trigger hyper-arousal for me are:

    _____

    _____

2. What I sense in my body when this happens is:

    _____

    _____

3. My behavior when I'm in this state is:

    _____

    _____

4. The thoughts I have are:

    _____

    _____

5. The emotions I tend to feel are:

    _____

    _____

Hypoarousal

1. The types of experiences, feelings, people, or environments that can trigger hypoarousal for me are:

    _____

    _____

2. What I sense in my body when this happens is:

    _____

    _____

3. My behavior when I'm in this state is:

_____

_____

4. The thoughts I have are:

_____

_____

5. The emotions I tend to feel are:

_____

_____

Optimum Arousal

1. The types of experiences, feelings, people, or environments that help me feel a balance of alertness and calmness are:

_____

_____

2. What I sense in my body when this happens is:

_____

_____

3. My behavior when I'm in this state is:

_____

_____

4. The thoughts I have are:

_____

_____

5. The emotions I tend to feel are:

_____

TITRATION AND THE WINDOW OF TOLERANCE

There is a broad range of challenging sensations or reactions you might experience as you begin to integrate your somatic awareness. Consider a few practices that you can do if/when you notice these.

1. **Sense of Overwhelm**
   Sit in a chair with your feet fully planted on the ground or stand with your spine extended. Slowly scan the environment and name objects in your field of vision. Bring your awareness to the sensations of groundedness that emerge through your connection to the earth and the experience of orienting.

2. **Shaking or Trembling**
   Take full, slow, mindful breaths. You can place a hand on your belly, the top of your head, or your chest if that feels good. You can also place a weighted blanket or comforter around yourself. Allow yourself to notice the sensations of the movement of shaking and also notice places you feel stable, solid, or still.

3. **Numbness or Disconnection**
   Gently squeeze your forearms with opposite hands. Gently rub, squeeze, or pat the tops of your thighs with your hands. Notice the sensations of your touch on your body.

4. **Accelerated Heart Rate**
   Move your attention away from your heart region by attending to the sensations in your feet and legs. Notice the sensations of groundedness and your connection with the floor or the chair.

5. **Collapsed in Body**
   If sitting in a chair, push your feet into the floor. If standing, push firmly against the wall with your arms fully extended and your head up. Feel the sensations of the movement.

PAUSING TO SUPPORT DOWN-REGULATION

Down-regulation is a practice of shifting your nervous system from sympathetic activation ("up-regulation") to parasympathetic engagement ("down-regulation"). Taking a pause when you notice the edges of activation allows you to teach your system how to down-regulate.

Self-directing your ability to down-regulate your nervous system is a foundational practice for healthy relationships. For example, research has shown that couples who are able to transition from high-arousal to low-arousal states show an increase in positive emotional behavior. Even if just one person in the couple is able to stay regulated, the other person has a better chance at becoming regulated.

1. When you notice sensations of sympathetic activation, hit the pause button and turn your attention inward to support self-soothing.

2. During the pause you can close your eyes, take a few deep breaths, bring your awareness to your feet on the floor, or notice the sensations of your back in the chair.

3. When you notice that you are activated, try saying to yourself, "I'm experiencing activation in this moment." If activation occurs when you are with another person, try saying, "I'm noticing that my nervous system is activated. I need a few moments to pause and breathe."

There is a direct relationship between language and the physiological arousal you experience in your body. During times of distress, you may have racing thoughts or speech that make it difficult to engage in supportive self-dialogue or constructive conversation with others. Labeling your emotion and articulating sensory awareness into language can help you slow down your thinking, more calmly articulate your feelings, and move through challenging situations.

Using simple descriptions, complete the following exercise using a real or hypothetical example. Return to follow the steps the next time you are triggered to create a dialogue of awareness with yourself.

1. When I am activated, the type of language I use (*Examples: critical or angry language, or statements that reflect extreme "black and white" thinking including words such as "always," "never," "disaster," or "ruined.") is:*

   _____

   _____

   _____

2. The resulting sensations in my body (*Examples: elevated heart rate, fluttering in my chest, stiffness in my jaw, etc.) are:*

   _____

   _____

   _____

3. Take a few slow, deep breaths. Direct your awareness to someplace inside your body that feels settled, at ease, or neutral. You can also use your gaze to look at something pleasant in your immediate environment.

4. Words of comfort I can say to myself (*Examples: I am safe. I can take my time, slow down, and wait until I feel calmer.) are:*

   _____

   _____

   _____

TAKING IN JUST A LITTLE

The following exercise will help you practice self-directing a titrated traumatic memory in order to manage activation. If at any time during this exercise you feel overwhelmed or flooded or you experience any feelings of "floatiness," remember that you can direct yourself back to grounded and resourced sensations in your body as you did in chapter 5.

1. Seat yourself in a comfortable position with something pleasant to look at in your field of vision that helps you feel calm.

2. Allow your eyes to close. Take a moment to find someplace inside your body that feels settled, pleasant, and at ease. Before working with a difficult memory we always want to be sure that we are starting from a resourced and grounded state.

3. Allow yourself to think of a short phrase that represents a traumatic memory or experience.

4. Notice what sensations or images you notice in response to the phrase. Allow yourself to take just a drop of any of the unpleasant sensations of activation. Hang out with the sensations for a few moments, until you start to feel like "that's enough."

5. As you close this practice, allow your gaze to rest on the object in your field of vision that is pleasant to look at from step 1. Let your gaze rest there and notice any shifts or changes that you feel inside your body.

Whether you are in the process of healing from relational trauma stemming from early development or you are processing a singular shock trauma, it can be helpful to create a timeline. Your body may not know that what happened in the past is over. An essential aspect of trauma processing is being able to notice the difference between then and now. A timeline can also help establish chronology and identify themes, which is helpful in contextualizing your past experience.

In the following chart, write whatever comes to mind about what you define as traumatic or upsetting memories, events, or stimuli you have experienced. In any circumstance there are often multiple survival impulses that are mobilized in the face of a threat. Identifying what feels unresolved is an opportunity for you to connect with any survival impulses you might have had, such as the part of you that wanted to run or the part of you that wished you'd stayed quiet instead of getting angry. Choose two to three words to title each note. Remember that selecting *just a few words* is a titration technique.

Age	Trauma Event Headline	What Feels Unresolved

DYNAMIC STRETCHING

Working directly with the body through movement is a helpful way to deepen your somatic awareness and support somatic therapy techniques. When it comes to stretching your body, there are two kinds of stretching: dynamic and static. Static stretching involves holding a position for a short period of time, without movement. Dynamic stretching is a movement-based form of stretching that uses the muscles to bring about a stretch. This practice will help you explore dynamic stretching in order to deepen your sensory experience of titration.

1. Find a comfortable position and clasp your hands together in front of your chest. Notice the sensations in your body.

2. Now, with your hands still clasped, extend your arms out in front of your chest and allow the backs of your hands to turn toward your body. Just go to *the edge* of where you feel the stretch and notice the sensations of the stretch. Sense into the experience of being at the edge without going farther into the stretch.

3. With your hands still clasped, release your arms and bring your hands back toward your chest. Notice that you just *pendulated* between the stretch and the release.

4. Repeat the movement and register the sensations in your arms and hands in the release position as relaxation and the sensations in the stretch position as tension.

5. Continue this movement at least four times.

6. As you end, take a few moments to reflect on what this experience was like for you.

Bilateral drawing is done with both hands. This exercise engages cross-hemisphere activity in the brain, which has been proven to promote trauma integration, self-regulation, and self-soothing.

Neuroplasticity is the brain's ability to change and adapt as a result of experience. When you create new positive associations or connect to resources in the present, you help the brain learn that you are no longer under the threat of the past. This exercise aims to orient to the here and now and slow down natural rhythms of breathing and heart rate.

For this exercise, use the space provided or a larger paper that you can tape down for greater ease when using both hands. Feel free to use oil pastels, chalk pastels, markers, colored pencils, crayons, or graphite sticks.

1. Select a headline from the timeline in the Creating a Timeline for Trauma exercise (page 92) as the prompt for the following activity. Write down the headline on a piece of paper or, if it feels safe, say it out loud and allow yourself to go just to the edge of the sensations of activation that arise.

2. Take a moment to sense into your body. You might follow a few cycles of breath, shake out your arms and hands, shimmy your chest—any movement impulse you are noticing your body wants to make.

3. The invitation is not to draw, but rather to allow your art materials to move on the page with your body. As the materials move, notice what rhythm feels good in your body. Play with different speeds and different movements that create different shapes. Explore asymmetrical movement and invite your hands to use the entire page.

4. Keep tracking the sensations and experiences of your body.

My Drawing

This exercise will allow you to experiment with grounding and pendulation, as well as a variety of titration skills you've learned in this chapter. Select another headline from your traumatic event timeline (page 92) or think of a recent experience that caused some activation. Complete the statements in the spaces provided. Note: Beginning from a resourced place in your body can help you stabilize if unpleasant sensations of activation arise.

A place that feels grounded or resourced in my body is:

_____

_____

_____

The sensations I notice in that area are:

_____

_____

_____

_____

The memory headline is:

_____

_____

_____

_____

When I write these words here or say these words out loud, what I notice in my body is:

_____

_____

_____

_____

The distance I want from this memory/experience that will allow me to experience a feeling of ease and space in my body is (*circle or write in the distance you want*):

- Across the room
- Across the street
- In another town
- Across the country
- On the other side of the globe
- In deep space
- Other: _____

The size I want to shrink this memory/experience down to that will allow me to experience a feeling of ease and space in my body is (*circle or write in the distance you want):*

- 3 feet
- 2 feet
- 1 foot
- 6 inches
- 3 inches and inside a glass jar
- Other: _____

Key Takeaways

Titration allows you to be present with just a little bit of activation at a time, which has the benefit of creating more space and allows for the innate, natural pendulation between parasympathetic and sympathetic activation to become established.

- One way that trauma is defined is "too much, too fast, too soon." Therefore, you want to create the opposite conditions: just a little bit, very slow, at just the right time.

- "The window of tolerance" is a term used to describe the zone of arousal in which a person is able to function most effectively. When you are within the optimal arousal zone, you are typically able to more readily receive, process, and integrate information and respond to the demands of everyday life without much difficulty.

- Titration skills include the use of distance, size, space, time, and support. Working with these features supports somatic awareness and also engages your creative capacities to expand your window of tolerance.

- Being intentional about your speech, such as word choice, simplified language, and attending to a slower pace of speech is a key titration and regulation skill.

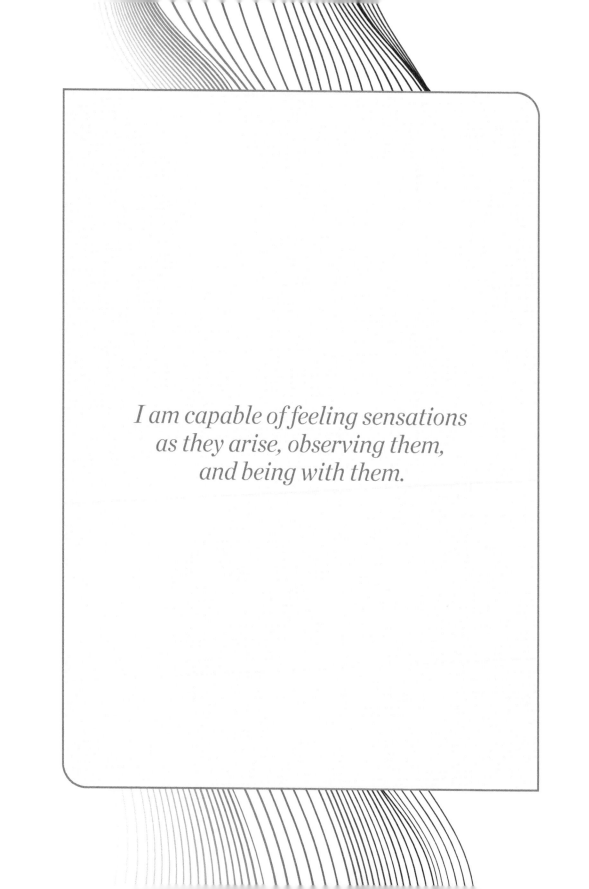

*I am capable of feeling sensations
as they arise, observing them,
and being with them.*

CHAPTER SEVEN

Recognizing How Trauma Leaves the Body with Sequencing Tools

In the regular course of life, there is a natural sequence of how you experience a situation, how you respond to it, and how you store the memory of it. When trauma occurs, this sequence is interrupted, making it difficult to process what happened and move on from it.

During a nontraumatic event, information arrives at a place in the brain known as the prefrontal cortex, which is responsible for processing information and then filing it away in another part of the brain called the hippocampus. During a trauma, however, this part of the brain goes off-line, which causes the trauma to become stuck in what is known as implicit memory (as if it is still happening) rather than moving into explicit memory (something that occurred in the past). Without the completion of this natural sequence, it's not just memories that become stuck—thoughts, behaviors, and sensations that you felt at the time of the trauma can also remain unprocessed and stay with you long after the event has occurred.

Sequencing techniques are designed to identify the stuck, frozen, or out-of-awareness parts of yourself that are still implicit and move them into awareness so that you can more fully heal.

Putting Sequencing into Practice

Imagine that you are out for a walk with your dog on a beautiful, sunny spring morning. Before you leave your home, you have a cup of coffee and a fresh blueberry muffin, make a phone call to a friend, grab your keys, and head out the door. As you move along the trail into the woods, you notice some daffodils beginning to peek their heads out of the earth, you see a hawk fly overhead, and you feel expansive and at peace. Then, totally unexpectedly, you hear your dog bark, and a brown bear appears on the path in front of you. Everything you were experiencing moments ago seems to be gone, and you are frozen under the threat of the bear.

In response to the threatening stimulus, your perception is focused on the source of the threat, and all the other aspects of your experience go off-line so that your system can prioritize survival. This narrow focus on survival is the reason that much of your implicit, or procedural, memory gets stored in the hippocampus outside of conscious awareness.

If you are able to widen your perceptual field, you will begin to create a sequence or timeline that brings more of your experience back into awareness and supports the release of other survival responses that may remain in your body. This somatic process helps you recognize that what you experienced is in the past and you are safe in the here and now, thus enhancing your capacity for self-regulation and increased capacity for life.

In Gestalt therapy there is a concept referred to as the "paradoxical theory of change." Simply put, *change occurs when we are able to be fully present with what is, not by avoiding or denying what is present, or attempting to be something else.* The more you begin to accept all the different feelings, sensations, thoughts, and aspects of your experience, the more whole you become. When you feel you need to eliminate or change a part of yourself, an almost automatic resistance is initiated inside of you. As you learn to meet all the parts of yourself with compassion and acceptance, these parts begin to introduce themselves to you and share with you how they came to exist. It's worth noting that accepting does not mean condoning what happened to you; rather, accepting the reality of what happened can help you begin to move beyond it. What parts of yourself, or of your experience, do you have the most difficulty accepting? How would it feel to meet these things with compassion and acceptance in order to heal?

_____

_____

_____

_____

_____

_____

_____

_____

_____

_____

_____

_____

_____

_____

An important part of trauma renegotiation is moving from fragmented or disowned parts of yourself into reintegrated wholeness. One way you can start to notice the different parts of yourself is by recognizing that everything that is whole is made up of parts. Think of your favorite food. If it's pizza, begin to notice all of the ingredients, or parts, that make up the pizza. Take your time to imaginatively explore the sensory experience of each ingredient by imagining their texture, shape, smell, and taste. What is it like to notice each part of the pizza? What is it like to be aware of the whole pie?

_____

_____

_____

_____

_____

_____

_____

Now think of the sensations inside your body. Focus on what it feels like to notice the sensation in your feet, your legs, your chest, and other body parts. Take a moment to notice what your body feels like as a whole entity. Describe your experience.

_____

_____

_____

_____

_____

_____

_____

_____

The word "emotion" is based on the Latin *emovere,* meaning "to move out." According to Dr. Jill Bolte Taylor, ninety seconds is all it takes to identify an emotion and observe it dissipate. When you learn to slow down and bring awareness to your somatic experience, you can learn to ride the waves of emotions. There is a sequence to a feeling when it moves through your body that mimics an actual wave: It wells up, swells, crests, washes over you, and then recedes into calm again. All emotions have equal value, as they are all part of the human experience. What do you notice about the sequence of a feeling when it moves through you?

CREATING SPACE AROUND DISCOMFORT

If you notice sensations of pain or discomfort in your body, you may notice your reactive or habitual behavior is to squirm, fidget, readjust, or resist. Next time you notice pain or discomfort, try pausing and observing the sensations instead of acting on them. Take a moment to allow your awareness to lightly touch upon the area of pain or discomfort. Take a deep breath and imagine creating space around the area in your body where you are noticing the pain or discomfort. Now allow your awareness to follow the impulse of the movement. Move slowly, with your full awareness on the sensations of the movement. What was your experience of slowing down the movement? What is your perceived difference between a more reactive or habitual movement in contrast to a slow and mindful movement?

OBSERVING A MOVEMENT SEQUENCE

The satisfaction cycle is a concept that comes from Bonnie Bainbridge Cohen's development of Body-Mind Centering (BMC). This influential work in the field of somatic therapy proposes that your early developmental movement patterns are essential to your sense of self, as well as how you view the world. Reconnecting with these movements can help support awareness of your body boundary, access healthy aggression, and allow you to satisfy your needs.

BMC includes five basic movements:

1. Yield

2. Push

3. Reach

4. Grasp

5. Pull

In each of the following movements, notice what muscles engage and notice the feeling of the movement. Bring your sensory awareness to your body. Move as slowly as you can in order to notice every micro-sensation of the movement. Take a moment to sit quietly and notice your experience after completing each movement.

1. Allow your body to **yield** by relaxing your muscles and feeling as though your body is softening. Keep your awareness of your body's connection to the floor as you yield.

2. **Push** against the floor or a wall.

3. **Reach** out in front of you toward something you can hold with your hands but that is currently beyond the reach of your arms.

4. Move toward the object and **grasp** it with your hands.

5. **Pull** the object toward your chest.

1. A trauma trigger is any stimulus that prompts an involuntary brain-body response from a previous traumatic experience. This involuntary response could be emotions such as fear, sadness, anger, and anxiety, or it could be a feeling of being overwhelmed. Or the response might be physiological symptoms, such as feeling frozen, a feeling of floatiness, an increased heart rate, nausea, dizziness, shaking, or sweating. Being triggered means that you reexperience symptoms of trauma when exposed to anything that is associated with the original trauma. The stimulus itself need not be frightening or traumatic and may be only indirectly or superficially reminiscent of an earlier traumatic incident; it might simply be a certain scent, tone of voice, or image.

2. The process of connecting the original traumatic experience with a trauma trigger is referred to as "traumatic coupling." When trauma is triggered, you move into an involuntary evolutionary response of hyperarousal (fight or flight) or hypoarousal (freeze) that can manifest in a variety of behavioral responses.

3. Move through the following table to identify your trigger and resources.

	Example	My Trigger and Resources
Name of trigger	*When someone yells at me*	
Touchstone event	*Memory of my dad yelling at me when I was seven years old*	
When I'm triggered, what I sense in my body is	*Tightness in my chest and fixedness in my eyes*	
As I track the sensation in my body, what happens next is	*Impulse to place my hand on my chest*	
Somatic resource	*Remember to find my feet on the floor and orient my gaze around the room*	
Social or spiritual resource	*Speaking with my sister or my connection to the natural world*	

DUAL AWARENESS

Dual awareness, a technique often used in somatic therapy to treat trauma, allows an individual to maintain awareness of two or more aspects of experience at the same time.

One consequence of traumatic stress is over-activation of the amygdala. The amygdala is the part of the brain that assists you in processing emotions, regulates how you respond to fear, and helps you create emotional memories. An overactive amygdala can mean that your brain has difficulty realizing the difference between a past threat and a present threat. This is why when you experience a trigger in the present, your amygdala responds the same way it did when you experienced the original trauma stimulus or event in the past.

A fundamental aspect of healing from trauma is allowing the past to touch the present. Dual awareness is a practice designed to establish that the present is safe and free of threat.

1. Find a comfortable seated position in a chair.

2. Notice the sensations on your body where the chair touches your upper legs and buttocks.

3. Now notice the contrasting sensations of the upper parts of your legs, which are exposed to the air and free of pressure.

4. Next, rest your awareness on the back and front of your body at the same time. Notice the contrasting sensations.

5. After a few minutes of exploring dual awareness, allow yourself to rest.

"Parts" work is a therapeutic process of attending to conflicts between various parts of yourself. An important aspect of parts work is to welcome in the multiplicity of your experience and to make space for any unresolved aspects of your experience that might block your efforts toward healing. The more space you can make for all of your parts, the more integrated you become.

For example, if you are working to address an experience of a violation to your physical body, you might be very in touch with an angry part, but if you don't also recognize the sad part of your experience, it can interfere with movement toward integration and healing.

Another aspect of parts integration may include behavior or movement. If for example, during the traumatic event you kicked and fought back, but another part of you wanted to freeze, then bringing that part into awareness is also important.

1. Begin by finding a quiet place where you can you relax. Close your eyes and turn your awareness inside your body. Start by saying "hello" to whatever sensations, thoughts, and feelings are present.

2. Give yourself some time to establish a resourced place inside your body where there is some sense of groundedness or ease.

3. Choose a traumatic memory that you'd like to work with and either think of a headline of the memory (such as one of those on your timeline in chapter 6 on page 92) or say the headline out loud.

4. Pause and notice any sensations of activation. Then say silently or out loud, "Hello, _____ part. I am aware of you." Allow yourself a few moments to sense the scared part, noticing the sensations, images, or emotions that may be associated with that part. Now, take a moment to open your eyes and fill out the first blank row in the table on the opposite page in relation to that part.

5. If you notice multiple parts (i.e., a scared part, a confused part, and a tight part), attend to one at a time, taking time to sense and be with each part, and complete the next rows in the table.

Part name	The sensations I noticed about that part	Write this statement in the space below: "Hello, _____part. You are welcome here."
Part 1:		
Part 2:		
Part 3:		

SPEAKING WITH YOUR PAST SELF

Working with a timeline is another crucial way in which you can move implicit ("still happening") traumatic memory to explicit ("happened in the past") memory. When you explore the timeline of your entire biography, as you did in chapter 6 (page 92), or work with a single memory, you allow parts of your somatic experience to come into awareness and develop your capacity to distinguish between the past and the present. One way you can create new neural connections and process traumatic memory is by allowing your present self to dialogue with your past self.

1. Identify a memory you'd like to work on.

2. Invite your adult, present self to ask the younger part of you to say a few words about their experience of the past.

3. Allow your younger self who experienced the traumatic event to respond. They might say, "It was so hard to be alone" or "I really needed someone to protect me."

4. Notice where you feel the younger part inside your body or notice what it feels like to make the expression from the past part.

5. Then allow your adult, present self to offer a statement of compassion and understanding. They might say, "That was really hard for you" or "I'm here to protect you now."

6. Take a few moments to notice your experience as you close.

If you notice that you are feeling activated, triggered, or dysregulated, invite the opposite quality. For instance, if you are tight, notice the part of you that is relaxed. If you feel scared, can you sense into the part of you that is brave? As you befriend and accept all the parts of yourself, you will notice that you'll begin to feel more integrated.

You can do this with movement and behavior as well. For instance, if you feel like curling up, you might follow the feeling of wanting to curl. Then you might sense into someplace inside your body that is opening, or wants to open, and follow this by finding a movement, such as opening your arms. If there is something inside you that feels frozen, you might explore the movement of running in place.

Think of a traumatic memory that you'd like to work with or refer to the timeline that you developed in chapter 6 (page 92) to support your work. Complete the following statements in your mind to deepen your awareness about your past experience. This will allow any sensations, behaviors, or emotional aspects of your experience to come more into awareness.

When _____ happened, I felt _____.
　　　　　　　　　　(memory)　　　　　　　　　　　　　　　　　　　　*(emotion)*

Part of me wanted to _____.
　　　　　　　　　　　　　　　　　　(behavior or image)

Another part of me felt _____ and wanted to _____.
　　　　　　　　　　　　　(emotion)　　　　　　　　　　*(behavior or image)*

Take a few moments afterward to notice how you feel before ending the practice.

This exercise will include an exploration of a theme in relation to trauma you have experienced. Common trauma themes might be abandonment, bullying, verbal abuse, medical procedures, or sexual abuse. The exercise can be activating for some people, so it is important to have the support of a therapist if you find it distressing or overwhelming.

1. Take some time to reflect on a theme you wish to explore.

2. When you have identified it, write down the first memory you have related to it in the table provided.

3. Add two subsequent memories.

4. Continue to fill out the table, noting your triggers, sensations, and emotions related to each memory.

5. As you work through the exercise, switch between each traumatic memory and a different, resourced memory you can recall from your life. This will help you feel more empowered about how you can resource yourself to feel more regulated if you encounter future experiences related to this theme in your life.

6. As you engage in this exercise, remember to use pendulation and grounding techniques, and take breaks whenever you start to feel sensations of overwhelm.

An example of how to complete the table is provided.

	Earliest memory	Second Memory	Most Recent Memory
Theme: *Other people's anger*	*Teacher yelling at me in second grade*	*Getting in trouble at camp*	*Boss expressed anger when email communication was late*
Triggers	*Loud, angry voices*	*Unfamiliar place*	*Boss's moods*
How dysregulating is the trigger on a scale of 1 to 10?	*8*	*2*	*8*
Sensations and location in the body	*Tight, prickling feeling in chest*	*Slightly alert in eyes and spine*	*Hot in my face and hollow in the pit of my stomach*
Emotion	*Scared*	*Alert*	*Ashamed*
Theme:			
Triggers			
How dysregulating is the trigger on a scale of 1 to 10?			
Sensations and location in the body			
Emotion			

One of the features of traumatic memory is that traumatic memories are stored implicitly (as if they are still happening) without explicit recall (as if they are in the past). Trauma is a felt sensory experience. Unprocessed traumatic memory is stored via the image (visual) and in the body (sensation) and not through the story (verbal). One of the benefits of art therapy in trauma processing is that there is direct access to the right hemisphere of the brain, where traumatic memories are stored. Making art does not rely on speaking and assists with the integration of sensory memories and explicit memory.

Choose a memory or event that you want to work with, something that you'd consider a 3 to 4 on a scale of 1 to 10 (see page 61). Begin by thinking of a headline that describes it (such as one of those on the timeline on page 92 in chapter 6). Notice any sensation, emotion, or experience inside your body that might feel a little incomplete, cloudy, or unfinished. Then use the blank space provided to draw whatever you visualize or feel in response to this.

You don't need to draw a lifelike depiction of the memory or event; rather, simply allow your energy to move onto the page through lines, shapes, and colors in a more abstract and free-form way. Do not worry about being a "good artist"—this process is about the experience, not the finished product. Sense into the feeling of the movement of your hand on the page.

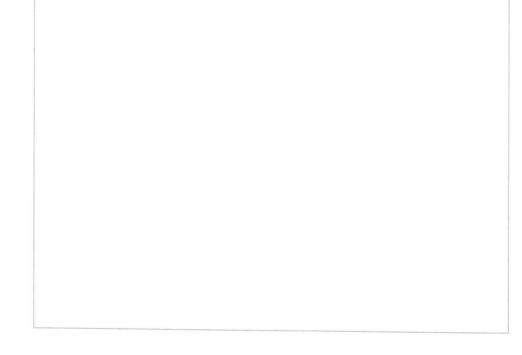

When you are finished drawing, take a moment to sense into your body and notice what sensations are present. What do you feel in your body after finishing?

_____

_____

_____

_____

_____

_____

_____

_____

_____

Is there a part of yourself or your experience that you are more aware of now? Describe it here.

_____

_____

_____

_____

_____

_____

_____

_____

_____

_____

_____

EXPLORING YOUR INNER LIFE USING PARTS

When you are working with your nervous system, you are working with different states of being. Your early attachment and developmental history, your genes, and the environments you were raised in all play a part in shaping your nervous system and your corresponding emotions, thoughts, and behavioral patterns.

Begin to practice noticing the different parts, or states of being, that are present at any given time. In any given moment you can practice dual awareness to be with multiple aspects of your experience simultaneously. This practice is a key technique to expanding your window of tolerance.

1. At any time throughout the day, take a moment to turn your awareness inside your body.

2. Imagine that you are alone, standing on a quiet small-town street, and whatever thoughts, sensations, emotions, or images are present are floats passing by in a parade. You are standing calmly and quietly while observing the different parts of you, with enough space and distance to feel regulated in your nervous system.

3. Take a few moments to track your experience and invite yourself to notice multiple aspects of it.

4. Then, try using "and" and "parts" language to support your expression of the whole of your experience. For example, "My feet feel really grounded, *and* there is some uncomfortable fluttering in my stomach. There is a *part* of me that feels overwhelmed *and* a *part* of me that knows this feeling won't last forever."

Key Takeaways

In somatic therapy, "sequencing" can refer to any aspect of traumatic experience that comes back in awareness, such as cognition, memory, felt-sense, or movement. Sequencing supports a deliberate processing of experience, allowing traumatic implicit memory to move into explicit memory.

Sequencing can involve any of the following concepts:

- Working with a timeline to bring more aspects of sensory experience into awareness.

- Working with somatic awareness to allow any movement or behavior to come into awareness and be expressed.

- Working with parts as a way to include the multiplicity of your experience and expand your window of tolerance.

- Dialoguing between different parts, such as your adult self to your younger self, in order to support discernment between past and present.

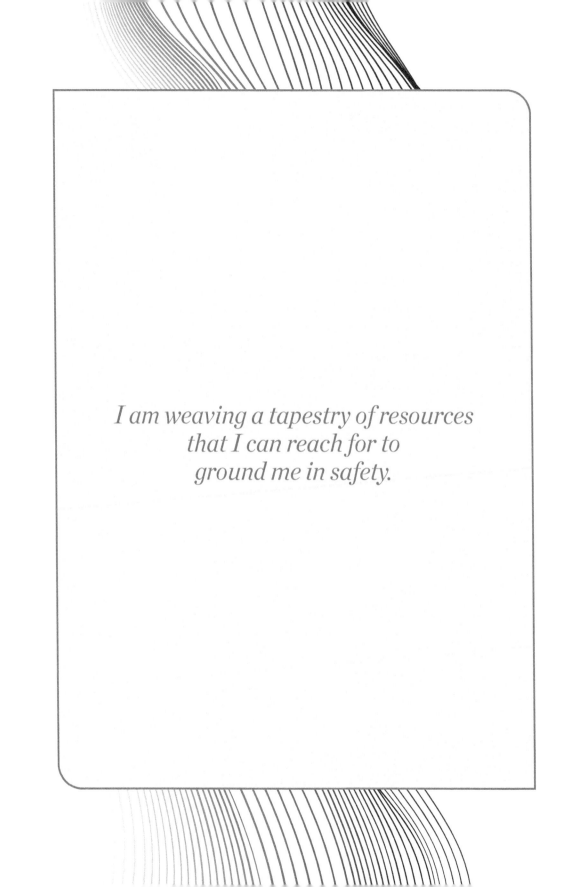

*I am weaving a tapestry of resources
that I can reach for to
ground me in safety.*

CHAPTER EIGHT

Creating Safe Spaces with Resourcing Techniques

A somatic resource is any tool or practice that engages the body to increase regulated nervous system states. Resourcing works to cultivate strategies that enable you to move out of activated states of fear or overwhelm and back into a sensory experience of safety in the present moment. Trauma and retraumatization (reliving the trauma of the experience) occurs when you do not have this sense of safety. You can cultivate internal resources through imagery, somatic tracking, breathing, movement, sound, or touch. And you can cultivate external resources through nature, animals, creativity, play, and safe interpersonal connection.

In this chapter, you will explore a variety of resourcing tools and practices to support your capacity for regulating your nervous system. Resource developing is a uniquely personal and creative process, so allow your connection to your body and your imagination to be the guide in your limitless capacity to identify, create, and build resources that support your feeling of safety.

Putting Resourcing into Practice

When you feel safe, you are more able to relax. When you are more able to relax, your "thinking brain" can come online and help you move implicit traumatic memory into explicit awareness. Additionally, when you feel safe, you are more able to be with the vulnerable parts of yourself, or the vulnerable sensations in your body. As you move forward, consider that the term "safe space" can refer to any resource that creates a felt-sense of safety.

When you are able to witness your vulnerable or uncomfortable somatic sensations, you have a window into your traumatic experiences and your resulting adaptive survival strategies. This awareness can illuminate the origin of your survival strategies and the reason you adopted them, and it can also invite you into witnessing the potentially hindering aspects of these continued responses or strategies.

Your ability to witness parts of yourself and your experiences, or to be witnessed by a therapist or other safe and trusted individual, is a fundamental aspect of self-understanding and trauma renegotiation. Being witnessed is an empowering acknowledgment of what you have lived through. Allowing yourself to observe what you feel in your body and acknowledge what you have survived is fundamental to your ability to understand that the past is over. Doing so allows you to recruit your life energy for living in the present.

Furthermore, compassionate witnessing helps you feel safe and relaxed with others so that you can safely and freely connect and explore in relationships. This promotes co-regulation, whereby you are able to help others cope with their own emotions by offering reassurance and comfort and can receive the same support in return.

Think about a place (real or imagined) that feels safe to you and brings you a feeling of comfort. Notice what elements create a feeling of safety for you. As you sense into the space and take in the details, notice what you feel in your body. Imagine that you are in your safe space, looking around, feeling the calm and peacefulness. Notice all the sensory details. If you don't feel safe, ask yourself gently what needs to change, then add or adapt the image to create more safety. This safe space is your creation. Keep visualizing and imagining it until you feel safe there. Feel free to go to your safe space when you are feeling dysregulated, going to sleep, or just wanting to have a few peaceful moments. What would you call this place? Describe the place below. What do you feel in your body when you are in your safe space?

CONNECTING WITH NATURE

Spending time in nature is simultaneously calming and inspiring. Research has shown that simply walking in nature can lower your risk for depression, reduce anxiety symptoms, improve mood, and increase cognitive functioning. Mindful, embodied connection with the natural world is a resource that you can reach for at any moment by going outside, looking out a window, or working with imagery. Embodiment in nature is about feeling your interconnectedness to all things and feeling that you are being held by something much larger than yourself. What are some of the connections you have to nature? What parts of the natural world make you feel connected, at ease, or inspired?

Trauma expert Dr. Bessel van der Kolk describes "being embodied" as the feeling of being present in your body and fully alive. When someone experiences a traumatic event, it can compromise their sensory abilities, including the five senses (smell, sound, sight, touch, and taste) and the ability to sense what is happening inside their bodies, such as a person's sense of pain and balance. This leads to a feeling of disembodiment or being detached from one's physical and emotional experiences.

Take a moment to sense into your body and write about what you observe in your internal experience. Then write about what you can observe outside of your body using your available senses. Doing so will help create feedback from your senses that allows your amygdala (page 109) to orient to safety, restoring your sense of embodiment.

One of the most painful aspects of trauma is often the invasion, intrusion, or collapse of boundaries with other people. Therefore, a key component of trauma is an ongoing feeling of threat to both physical and emotional safety. Not knowing where "I" end and the "other" begins can create disorganization, chaos, and confusion in a person's inner world. To heal, you must attend to building and embodying your boundaries.

Do you have a sense of your own personal space that exists beyond the surface of your skin? What happens when someone is too close?

_____

_____

_____

_____

_____

_____

_____

What is a distance that feels safe for your body? Are there any other boundaries around physical space or your body that you feel are important?

_____

_____

_____

_____

_____

_____

_____

VISUALIZING A NURTURING FIGURE

Trauma can affect your ability to trust others and feel loved and cared for. One resource you can use to restore these capacities is to visualize a nurturing figure.

1. Find a comfortable position and close your eyes.

2. Imagine a person, animal, or any other symbol that carries a nurturing quality—somebody or something that makes you feel loved and cared for. This figure can be fictional or real.

3. Take a moment to visualize your nurturing figure. Notice the somatic sensations and experience as you visualize the nurturer.

4. Now find a movement or gesture that expresses the feeling of being nurtured. You might wrap your arms tightly around your body, place a hand lovingly to your heart, or place a hand tenderly on your face.

5. Allow yourself to feel loved and cared for by this figure.

When you are finished visualizing, feel free to draw, paint, or collage an image of this nurturing figure on a separate piece of paper that you can refer to when needed.

VISUALIZING A PROTECTOR FIGURE

While a nurturing figure provides you with love and care, you can think of a protector figure as a loyal and fearless security guard who keeps you safe from any threatening stimulus you may encounter. Visualizing this figure can help you shift out of overwhelming emotions and feel safer and more empowered.

1. Find a comfortable position and close your eyes.

2. Begin to invite in an image of a protective figure—a person, animal, or symbol that can offer ferocious protection from any threatening stimulus you might encounter.

3. As you call in your protective figure image, notice the sensations in your body. Notice the feelings and positive thoughts associated with the image.

4. Now find a movement or gesture that expresses the feeling of being protected. You might make your hands into claws or open your jaw and roar like a lion.

When you are finished, feel free to draw, paint, or collage an image of this protective figure on a separate piece of paper that you can refer to when needed.

We can't say yes if we can't say no. Many people struggle with saying no or setting limits. The fear or anxiety of saying no often stems from an urge to avoid conflict or confrontation. Another reason some people tend to worry about saying no is that they want to please others or not disappoint others. However, when you don't have access to saying no, you disrupt the most important safe space you have: your body. Practicing saying no in the safety and comfort of your own space is great rehearsal so that when you have a real-life opportunity, the word and the feeling of saying it will come more easily to you.

1. Say "no" out loud several times and notice your inner sensations. Describe your breath, gestures, movements, and emotional experience.

   _____

   _____

   _____

   _____

2. List three situations in which you would have liked to have said no but didn't or couldn't. Next to each one, make note of what stopped you from saying no.

   _____

   _____

   _____

   _____

3. Select one of the situations in which you'd like to say no in the future and practice saying it out loud. Notice your feelings, movements, breath, and tone of voice. Write down what you observe. Note: You might bring in your body-boundary awareness, protectors, safe space, or any other resources that support your feeling of safety as you say no.

   _____

   _____

   _____

   _____

Your access to your somatic experience is the grounding for sensing if you want to move toward something or away from something. Saying yes with your full awareness can be an empowering experience.

Practice saying yes and complete the following prompts to record your experience strengthening your awareness.

1. Say "yes" out loud several times and notice your somatic experience. Describe your breath, gestures, movements, and emotional experience.

    _____

    _____

    _____

2. List three situations in which you would have liked to have said yes but didn't or couldn't. Next to each one, make note of what stopped you from saying yes.

    _____

    _____

    _____

3. List three situations in which you'd like to be able to say yes in the future.

    _____

    _____

    _____

4. Select one of the situations in which you'd like to say yes in the future and practice saying it out loud. Notice your feelings, movements, breath, and tone of voice. Write down what you observe.

    _____

    _____

    _____

This is a practice you can do if you notice sensations of dysregulation after encountering a trigger. You can also use this practice to work with events from your trauma timeline on page 92.

1. Find a comfortable seated position.

2. Begin by grounding yourself in the present moment. Feel your feet firmly on the floor and the support of the chair beneath your body.

3. Think of a recent moment when you felt resourced. Visualize yourself as capable, wise, strong, and protected. Notice the sensations in your body as you visualize this image.

4. Lean forward very slowly in your chair and have the here-and-now resourced part of yourself reach into the past and grab the version of yourself who experienced the traumatic event. Allow your arms to open and grab onto the vulnerable, scared part of you. Now close your arms in toward your chest and pull the past part of you into the resourced present.

5. Give yourself time to observe what you notice and simply feel what you feel.

6. Now look around the room. Feel your feet on the floor. Give yourself time to orient to the present moment.

7. Sense into your body for any remaining sensations of activation. If you still notice sensations of activation, reach back into the past and grab any remaining parts of you that are still there.

8. Imagine hugging the past version of yourself. Tell them that they are safe and protected by you in the present. Now rest.

"Trigger" is a term used to refer to the stimulus that kicks off physiological activation. Though it isn't clear exactly how triggers are formed, some researchers posit that the brain stores memories from a traumatic event differently from memories of nontraumatic events. When you have a traumatic experience, your brain and body capture the associated sensory stimulus at the time of the event, also known as "coupling," and these stimuli can become associated with the threatening experience. For example, if you saw a blue house at the time you were chased by a dog, you may have a negative physiological reaction whenever you see a blue house.

Think of a trigger as a well-meaning alarm system from your body to alert you to a real or perceived threat. The ability to map out your triggers can help you understand what information your body is attempting to offer you. It can be helpful to have a plan so that when you feel activated, you have a way you can call in resources. Answer the following questions to think through your own plan.

1.   What trigger do you wish to explore? *(Example: When my partner forgets something I have said before.)*

     _____

     _____

     _____

     _____

     _____

2.   What sensations do you typically experience when triggered? *(Example: Expanding through my chest, prickling sensation in my neck.)*

     _____

     _____

     _____

     _____

     _____

     _____

3. What feelings typically arise when you are triggered? *(Example: Primary feeling is fear, secondary feeling is anger.)*

_____

_____

_____

_____

4. How do you usually react when triggered? *(Example: I become critical and accuse them of forgetting.)*

_____

_____

_____

_____

5. What is an internal resource that you can reach for? *(Example: Pausing, taking a deep breath, feeling my feet on the floor.)*

_____

_____

_____

_____

6. What is an external resource that you can reach for? *(Example: I can lean on my partner if I respond calmly, remind them of my sensitivity around the issue, and ask for their support.)*

_____

_____

_____

_____

SENSING INWARD

You are likely aware of your available senses, but you may not be as aware of interoception, a lesser-known sense that helps you feel and understand what is happening inside of your body.

Engaging in movement can help wake up this somatic sensation to help you feel more present and embodied. The following practice is a great way to achieve this.

1. Face a wall and stand about a foot or so away from it with your legs shoulder-distance apart and feet planted firmly on the floor.

2. Bend your knees, keep your arms close to your body, and push into the wall with your hands using the strength of your arms.

3. Sense into the feeling of your back muscles as you push with your hands and arms. Hold a dual awareness of the engagement in your legs and your arms.

4. Push for as long as your body wants and then let go.

5. Notice the sensations of release or relaxation after you stop pushing while still keeping your awareness of being connected to the floor.

6. Do this a few times. Then rest.

STEERING THE BOAT

When you are experiencing activation in your nervous system, you might think of your nervous system as a sailboat that's gone off course. As the captain of the boat, you want to assist bringing it back to its preferred path. The following practice allows you to sense into feeling off-center before rebalancing yourself, helping you to feel like a more capable captain of your felt experience.

1. Stand in place and allow your eyes to gaze down at the floor in front of you.

2. Imagine a midline in the center of your body, as if there were a string that went down the front of your body.

3. Now, very slowly, tip a little to one side and notice the feeling of being off-center of the midline. Notice the feeling of that movement and the sensations you are aware of in your body.

4. Now, very slowly, bring yourself back to center. Notice the feeling of that movement and the corresponding sensations that you are aware of in your body.

5. Do this a few times, moving very slowly so that you can sense the movement. Then rest.

Every moment of the day, your somatic state is changing in response to the thoughts in your head as well as the stimuli in your environment. Just like sensory stimuli, the thoughts you have and how you speak to yourself affect how you feel in your body and your sense of yourself in the world.

Those who have experienced trauma tend to report higher levels of shame and self-critical thoughts, which in turn can negatively affect their somatic experience. Research has shown that affirmations trigger the reward centers of the brain known to lessen pain and maintain balance when threatened. You can use the below sample affirmations to identify your somatic experience, or you can bring your creativity to the process of writing your own affirmations.

Resilience Affirmation

My affirmation (Example: I survived, and I am here today.):

_____

_____

What I feel in my body as I say this is:

_____

_____

The image that comes to mind is:

_____

Nurturing Affirmation

My affirmation (Example: Nothing feels better than caring for myself.):

_____

_____

What I feel in my body as I say this is:

_____

_____

The image that comes to mind is:

_____

Protective Affirmation

My affirmation (Example: I can visualize a protective figure to give me strength.):

_____

_____

What I feel in my body as I say this is:

_____

_____

The image that comes to mind is:

_____

Body-Boundary Affirmation

My affirmation (Example: I decide who comes into my space. I am firm in my ability to say yes or no.):

_____

_____

What I feel in my body as I say this is:

_____

_____

The image that comes to mind is:

_____

Key Takeaways

A somatic resource is any tool or practice that engages the body to increase regulated nervous system states. Resourcing works to cultivate strategies that enable you to move out of activated states of fear or overwhelm and back into a sensory experience of safety in the present moment. Resource developing is a uniquely personal and creative process; however, here are a few common resourcing practices in somatic therapy:

- Internal resources are generated from your ability to direct your awareness to a place inside of your body that feels safe and grounded, which you can do through imagery, somatic tracking, breathing, movement, sound, or touch.

- External resources can include the natural world, beloved animals from your life, creativity, play, and safe interpersonal connection.

- You can create safe spaces—real or imagined places where you can establish regulated safety in your body.

- Nurturing or protective figures that support a feeling of safety can be a resource.

- Establishing and practicing body boundaries can be a resource, as well as practicing saying yes and no.

- Verbal affirmations can be a resource.

A Final Note

Congratulations on completing this somatic therapy and embodiment journey! I hope these pages have provided you with some fundamental nervous system education, and I hope you'll use these practices for support as you continue to develop your relationship with your body and heal from any trauma you have experienced. The more you learn to listen to the wisdom of your body, the more you can cultivate a sensitive, compassionate, and attentive relationship with your body.

The benefits of living an embodied life extend far beyond healing from traumatic experiences. Living an embodied life means experiencing the wholeness of life. This includes trusting in the intuitive wisdom that arises from your body about what you need and want, having boundary confidence and attunement, feeling empowered to live in alignment with your values, having greater self-awareness and insight, having an increased capacity for intimacy and connection with others, and having an increased capacity to live in the present moment.

I wish you well as you continue to cultivate an embodied life, and I am grateful to have had a chance to walk alongside you for a while.

Resources

Books

Trauma and Memory: Brain and Body in a Search for the Living Past: A Practical Guide for Understanding and Working with Traumatic Memory by Peter A. Levine

Healing Trauma: A Pioneering Program for Restoring the Wisdom of Your Body by Peter A. Levine

The Wisdom of Your Body: Finding Healing, Wholeness, and Connection Through Embodied Living by Hillary L. McBride

Moving Beyond Trauma: The Roadmap to Healing from Your Past and Living with Ease and Vitality by Ilene Smith

Widen the Window: Training Your Brain and Body to Thrive During Stress and Recover from Trauma by Elizabeth A. Stanley

The Body Keeps the Score: Brain, Mind, and Body in the Healing of Trauma by Bessel A. van der Kolk

Organizations

Somatic Experiencing International is a nonprofit 501c3 based on the teaching of Dr. Peter Levine that's dedicated to transforming lives through healing | instagram.com /somaticexperiencingint/

Podcasts

The Embodiment Podcast: Conversational explorations of all things embodied, including yoga, trauma, dance, bodywork, culture, etc. | embodimentunlimited.com/podcast/

"This Conversation Will Change How You Think About Trauma." *The Ezra Klein Show* | podcasts.apple.com/us/podcast/this-conversation-will-change-how-you-think-abouttrauma /id1548604447?i=1000532955898

The Healing Trauma Podcast: Somatic Experiencing with Joshua Sylvae | podcasts.apple .com/gb/podcast/somatic-experiencing-with-joshua-sylvae/id1444361384?i =1000555390645

Websites

"What is Pendulation in Somatic Experiencing with Peter A. Levine." Somatic Experiencing International | youtube.com/watch?v=LiXOMLoDm68

"The Body Keeps the Score." The School of Life | youtube.com/watch?v=QSCXyYuT2rE

Irene Lyons is a nervous system specialist and somatic neuroplasticity expert. She offers free content and courses to support nervous system education and healing | irenelyon.com

"Healing the Nervous System from Trauma: Somatic Experiencing Video." Therapy in a Nutshell | youtube.com/watch?v=dMmEdsuPRiU

"Turn off Anxiety in Your Nervous System: 4 Ways to Turn on the Parasympathetic Response." Therapy in a Nutshell | youtube.com/watch?v=FPH5CFSmYEU

"Dr. Stephen Porges: What is the Polyvagal Theory." PsychAlive | youtube.com/watch?v=ec3AUMDjtKQ

"15-Minute Body Scan Meditation Somatic Awareness Guided Meditation, Mind-Body Healing." American Academy of Mind-Body Healing | youtube.com/watch?v=KE9N3ukCYdw

References

Bainbridge Cohen, Bonnie, Lisa Nelson, and Nancy Stark Smith. *Sensing, Feeling, and Action: The Experiential Anatomy of Body-Mind Centering.* Northampton, MA: Contact Editions, 1993.

Boyd, Jenna E., Ruth A. Lanius, and Margaret C. McKinnon. "Mindfulness-Based Treatments for Posttraumatic Stress Disorder: A Review of the Treatment Literature and Neurobiological Evidence." *Journal of Psychiatry and Neuroscience* 43, no. 1 (January 2018): 7–25. doi:10.1503/jpn.170021.

Campbell, Melissa, Kathleen P. Decker, Kerry Kruk, and Sarah P. Deaver. "Art Therapy and Cognitive Processing Therapy for Combat-Related PTSD: A Randomized Controlled Trial." Art Therapy 33, no. 4 (October 2016): 169–177. doi: 10.1080/07421656.2016.1226643.

Cascio, Christopher N., Matthew Brook O'Donnell, Francis J. Tinney, Matthew D. Lieberman, Shelley E. Taylor, Victor J. Stretcher, and Emily B. Falk. "Self-Affirmation Activates Brain Systems Associated with Self-Related Processing and Reward and Is Reinforced by Future Orientation." *Social Cognitive and Affective Neuroscience* 11, no. 14 (April 2016):621–9. doi: 10.1093/scan/nsv136.

Heitzler, Morit. "Broken Boundaries, Invaded Territories: The Challenges of Containment in Trauma Work." *International Body Psychotherapy Journal* (March 2013): 28–41.

Levine, Peter A. *In An Unspoken Voice.* Berkeley, CA: North Atlantic Books, 2010.

Levine, Peter A. *Trauma and Memory: Brain and Body in a Search for the Living Past: A Practical Guide for Understanding and Working with Traumatic Memory.* Berkeley, CA: North Atlantic Books, 2015.

LoPreseti, Robert. "A Ritual for Resolving Chronic, Habitual, and Pathological Implicit Memory and Emotional Disorders, Including Grief and Trauma." *Body Psychotherapy Journal* 10, no. 2 (2011): 32–52.

Malchiodi, C. "Art Therapy and the Brain." In C. Malchiodi (Ed.), *Handbook of Art Therapy.* New York: Guilford, 2003, pp 17–26.

Ogden, Pat, and Janina Fisher. *Sensorimotor Psychotherapy: Intervention and for Trauma and Attachment.* New York: W. W. Norton & Company, 2015.

Oschman, James L., Gaétan Chevalier, and Richard Brown. "The Effects of Grounding (Earthing) on Inflammation, the Immune Response, Wound Healing, and Prevention and Treatment of Chronic Inflammatory and Autoimmune Disease." *Journal of Inflammation Research* 8 (March 2015): 83–96. doi:10.2147/JIR.S69656.

Osterweis, Marian, and Arthur Kleinman. *Pain and Disability: Clinical, Behavioral, and Public Policy Perspectives.* Washington, DC: National Academies Press, 1987.

Papathanassoglou, Elizabeth D. E., and Meropi D. A. Mpouzika. "Interpersonal Touch: Physiological Effects in Critical Care." *Biological Research for Nursing* 14, no. 4 (October 2012): 431–43. doi:10.1177/1099800412451312.

Parnell, Laura. *Attachment-Focused EMDR: Healing Relational Trauma.* New York: W.W. Norton & Company, 2013.

Payne, Peter, Peter Levine, and Mardi. A. Crane-Godreau. "Somatic Experiencing: Using Interoception and Proprioception as Core Elements of Trauma Therapy." *Frontiers in Psychology* 6 (February 2015): 93. doi:10.3389/fpsyg.2015.00093.

Rosenberg, Stanley. *Accessing the Healing Power of the Vagus Nerve: Self-Help Exercises for Anxiety, Depression, Trauma, and Autism.* Berkeley, CA: North Atlantic Books, 2017.

Shapiro, Robin. *Easy Ego State Interventions.* New York: W.W. Norton and Company, 2016.

van der Kolk, Bessel A. *The Body Keeps the Score: Brain, Mind, and Body in the Healing of Trauma.* New York: Penguin Publishing Group, 2015.

Yuan, Joyce. W., Megan McCarthy, Sarah R. Holley, and Robert W. Levenson. "Physiological Down-Regulation and Positive Emotion in Marital Interaction." Emotion 10, no. 4 (August 2010): 467–74. doi:10.1037/a0018699.

Index

A

Abdominal breathing, 31
Activation observation, 60
Affirmations
  creating safety with, 136–137
  defined, 21
  grounding, 54
Anxiety, somatic therapy for, 7
Art therapy, 116–117
Autonomic nervous system, 4, 5, 12

B

Belly breathing, 31
Bilateral drawing, 94–95
Body awareness
  about, 15, 23, 37
  beach imagery exercise, 35
  belly breathing, 31
  body scanning, 27
  physical sensations in the
    body, 29, 32
  progressive muscle
    relaxation, 30
  relaxation in the body, 17, 23, 25
  stepping-stones exercise, 28
  stress in the body, 26
  tension in the body, 17, 23
Body-Mind Centering (BMC), 107
Body scanning, 27
Body therapy, 4
Bottom-up therapy, 4
Boundary setting, 126
Brach, Tara, 74

Breathing exercises
  belly breathing, 31
  ocean rhythm breathing, 35

C

Change, accepting, 103
Character Analysis (Reich), 4
Chronic pain, 7–8, 13
Cohen, Bonnie Bainbridge, 107
Complex post-traumatic stress disorder
    (C-PTSD), 6–7
Crown technique, 45

D

Depression, somatic therapy for, 7
Discomfort, creating space
    around, 106
Down-regulation, 89
Dual awareness, 109
Dynamic stretching, 93

E

Earth, connection with, 41, 46
Embodiment, 125
Emotional trauma, 13

F

"Felt-sense" concept, 4
Fight, flight, freeze, or fawn
    response, 5, 9
5-4-3-2-1 grounding technique, 52–53
Flooding, emotional, 82

T

Taylor, Jill Bolte, 105
Tension
  language for, 36
  melting, 33
  observing in the body, 17, 23
Titration
  about, 16, 79–80, 98
  activation management exercise, 91
  bilateral drawing, 94–95
  distancing exercise, 83, 96–97
  down-regulation, 89
  dynamic stretching, 93
  experience shrinking, 84, 96–97
  just a drop concept, 82
  just the edge concept, 81
  regulation language, 90
  trauma timeline, 92
  window of tolerance, 85–88
Tolle, Eckhart, 43
Touch, 14
Tracking, 23, 34, 36
Trauma
  emotional, 13
  healing from, 8–9

implicit vs. explicit memory of, 15
  mind-body connection, 8
  physical, 13
  somatic therapy and, 5–7
  timeline for, 92
  triggers, 108, 132–133
  understanding, 12
Traumatic coupling, 108
Triggers, 108, 132–133

V

Vagus nerve, 47
van der Kolk, Bessel, 5, 8, 125
Visualization. *See also* Imagery
  of a nurturing figure, 127
  of a protector figure, 128

W

Water grounding, 48
Wholeness, 104
Window of tolerance, 12, 68, 72–73, 76
    85–88

Y

"Yes!" saying, 130
Yoga, 50

Acknowledgments

First and foremost, I would like to thank my Somatic Experiencing mentor and teacher, Larry Iannotti. Thank you for being a source of wisdom, comfort, and support in helping me come back home to my body.

Thank you to my clients, who reveal to me every day the extraordinary resilience of the human spirit.

Thank you to the entire Gestalt Associates for Psychotherapy community for being a home of comfort, growth, and authentic connection.

Thank you to my family and friends for their support of this project. Thank you to Yoon Im Kane and Alicia Muñoz for their writing mentorship. Thank you to Jennifer Byxbee, Rob York, Bill Barclay, Jennifer Bunin, Lindsay Clark, and Blake Blankenbecler—your limitless encouragement, collegial support, and friendship are a cherished wellspring.

In particular, thank you to my husband, Keith Elijah Fasciani. You have made this life for me.

About the Author

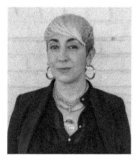 **Jordan Dann, LP,** is a dynamic psychoanalyst and educator. Jordan has advanced training as a Gestalt therapist, Somatic Experiencing Practitioner, and Imago Relationship Therapist, along with many years of coaching and directing actors. Her innovative approach helps individuals and couples become more embodied and connected. She is a nationally certified and New York State–licensed psychoanalyst in private practice in New York City and serves as an associate faculty member for the Gestalt Associates for Psychotherapy. You can follow her on Instagram @jordandann.

Printed in the USA
CPSIA information can be obtained
at www.ICGtesting.com
CBHW041157090424
6568CB00007B/65

9 781685 393779